THE PRIVATE PRACTICE MBA

The Rise of the Medpreneur

Dr. Joseph Simon

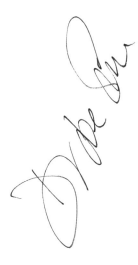

THE PRIVATE PRACTICE MBA
The Rise of the Medpreneur
By Dr. Joseph Simon
Copyright © 2015 Dr. Joseph Simon

For my Girls: Sophia & Lily

Thanks for teaching me to never take myself too seriously

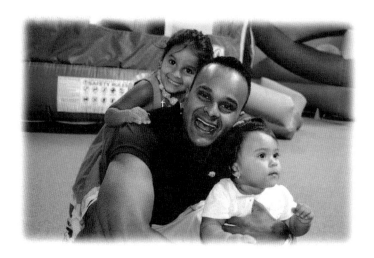

Table of Contents

THE PRIVATE PRACTICE MBA

Introduction

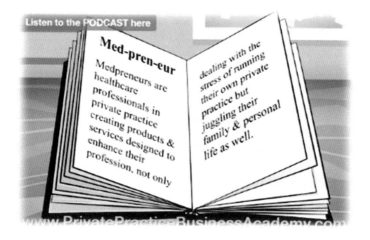

"The best time to plant a tree was 20 years ago. The

second best time is now."

– Chinese proverb.

I'm Dr. Joe Simon, and in a nutshell, I love seeing people thrive. That's why I do what I do, and that's why I've written this book. I'm a practitioner, just like you are, or maybe soon will be. I trained as a physical therapist, so it's an area I always keep an especially

1

close eye on. But this book is about all Medpreneurs, of course, and I'm more than confident that the lessons I've put forward here will apply to all health care practitioners who are part of this ever-growing and lucrative trend of the cash-based practice.

What is a Medpreneur? In brief, it's just what it sounds like—a combination of a medical practitioner and an entrepreneur. The word is out there gaining traction, and it's what I want you to be. I use the word because it encompasses many types of medical practice into one word—and because the advice I give you regarding it should apply equally to PT-preneurs, dental-preneurs, and all other permutations.

In the last few years, we've seen slow but significant and inevitable changes in the way the whole healthcare field works. Health insurance, as I'm sure you've experienced, has gone from something both doctors and patients found steady and reliable, to a huge source of uncertainty for everyone. A lot of doctors are finding the ways they have always used to get patients are now not working, and they are trying to figure out what to do about it. A lot of older doctors are closing clinics and practices because they are finding that patients are no longer coming in after being referred by internists. With more and more people turning to the internet to diagnose themselves, many are choosing to forgo a visit to their general practitioner to instead find a specialist.

The average person finds these specialists via Google and recommendations from friends, instead of through traditional referrals. For the huge number of doctors with no online presence, this means they are now essentially invisible. It's easy to try to place blame elsewhere—on health insurance, republicans, democrats, Obama. That's not where the fault lies.

The real cause is the fact that most doctors are not trained to be businesspeople, so they don't know how to be entrepreneurs. And the ones that do have a huge edge. The new crop of doctors coming out of medical programs nationwide understand the system is changing. They know people find their information online now, because that's what they themselves do. But they still need to compete as businesspeople in a business world, without ever having received business training. These new medical entrepreneurs are ready to start businesses today, and some are realizing that it can essentially be done with nothing more than a cell phone and a treatment table. Some people are even practicing telemedicine over Skype. They're starting to share their knowledge instantaneously over the Internet.

They're the Medpreneurs. They're what's taking over medicine. They're the medical professionals starting their businesses with nothing down and little more than an internet connection and a laptop. They're the future, and you can become one of them. If you don't, you'll be competing against them instead—and that's a losing battle. That doesn't mean you have to be just starting in order to succeed. On the contrary, established practices have an advantage in that they already have cash flow—not to mention staff, support, and brick-and-mortar locations. What they have to fight against is the idea that they might be too big to move; their maneuverability will always be slower than that of a one-person practice.

Even the word "entrepreneur" is growing. A few years ago, people would hear "entrepreneur" and think,

"Oh. You must be unemployed." Now the word is looked on with reverence. It means you've taken risks and you know how to handle things. And this tidal wave in modern culture is going to be one that we can ride using the expertise taught by my Private Practice Business Academy.

I coach clients every day who are working on starting their own practice, or who have one already but want help making it grow or preventing it from failing. I started because it was something I had a passion and a talent for, and I've only become better at it. I've helped over 13,000 practitioners to date, and I keep doing it because it's what I love. I love the marketing and sales aspects, and I love the interpersonal aspect even more. I know this is what I'm good at, and I know what you are good at. And I know what it is you need to work on if you want to make your practice explode with success in the coming years.

As a physical therapist myself, that's where most of my experience is. But if you're a psychiatrist, or an acupuncturist, or a dentist, or something else, don't put this book down. As I've been saying, we're all in the same business. We all want to be experts in bringing clients in through the door. And as you grow your practice, continuing to do that will be your cornerstone.

As I take you through the journey of this book, I want to give you a lot of my own advice on starting, running, growing, and promoting a cash-based, out-of-network private practice. And I'm also going to supplement that knowledge with examples and stories of other practitioners whom I know and have dealt with. As you'll see, a huge key to success in the private practice world is in finding your niche, and a person's niche is personal and unique enough that I want you to know how other people like you and me have found theirs.

I'd like to think of this book as part of an education. Some things you pay for to make yourself better, and education tends to be one of them. What I am giving you here is an education on how to make your practice better. This book isn't the only step, because it wouldn't be possible to teach everything in one book. Your effort, time, and monetary investment will determine how well-educated you become in regards to running your practice. But I try to give away as many strategies as possible, and I'm always here in my coaching capacity to help people who want to implement these strategies.

Chapter One

The Medpreneur Within

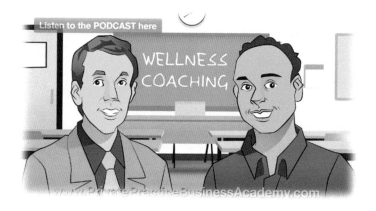

"Choose a job that you like, and you will never have to

work a day in your life."

– Confucius

Let me tell you about myself. I want you to know who this advice is coming from. And hey, you might even find some parts of my story inspiring once you know how I arrived where I am.

When I graduated in 2001, having trained as a doctor of physical therapy, I did what most physical therapists do immediately upon earning their degrees. I said to myself, "I need to get a job so I can pay off my student loans." Now, I know what you may be thinking. *'The guy's a physical therapist! He can get a job anywhere he wants!'* Well, that is part of the beauty of my specialty, but the downside of it is that in most cases, once you get hired, you are going to be pigeonholed doing the same thing for the next ten to twenty years, treating maybe twenty to forty patients a day depending on where you work. Some of you know it already, but let me tell you: that can be exhausting.

Sometimes, you work for fantastic people, and you think it's great. Other times, frankly, you work for absolute idiots. Unfortunately, the latter tended to be truer for me. I worked with some great people, but I worked with an even greater number who simply made me furious. Because of that, I realized I had more of an entrepreneurial drive than most of my associates. And to be honest, when I first started in the medical community there weren't that many entrepreneurs around. At that time, insurance companies determined what we got paid, and that was basically it.

Steps to My Own Practice

When I started my journey as an entrepreneur, I made thousands of mistakes. I started my own practice, and I kept my day job at the time because I had bills and rent to pay. I was still young enough that I wanted to be able to go out and enjoy life. So my biggest goal as an entrepreneur was to be able to pay for my vacations and maybe some of the little extra comforts in life. Now, that's not necessarily a bleak picture, I know. I was making extra money to vacation and enjoy myself, while most people are just trying to get enough money together to pay the bills. But I soon realized that was just the tip of the iceberg. It became quite clear to me that I could make more money if I was in business for myself, with my own practice, than I ever could working for somebody else.

When you're working for someone else, it can be dangerously easy to be pulled down by a lack of upward mobility. And for us in the medical field, it can be very easy to become addicted to the fact that we're making good money. But no matter how well you happen to be doing, if you're somebody's employee, your real task is to make money for your boss rather than yourself. The message that's being sent to you, directly or indirectly, is "You need to see more people so you can pay the bills, and pay your salary." They don't care how stressful it is—the more people you see, the more money they make.

But eventually, the burnout factor is going to kick in, and that is not something you can quantify on a time sheet. With time, it happened to me. I was making good money, and all I needed was a little bit extra. But I started realizing I couldn't go on with things as they were. Every profession has its own "lifespan," as I like to call it. We physical therapists don't spend most of our time behind desks; we're using our bodies a lot in our work. So our lifespan in terms of the time before our hands or back or something else starts to give out isn't always very long. In healthcare fields, it tends to be about ten years. In dentists or podiatrists, the lower back starts to break down. For us physical therapists, it's the hands. As I saw that ten-year mark beckoning to me down the road, I thought to myself, "I have to figure something out."

I had this all in the back of my head, and I eventually got to the point where I realized I wanted to make some extra money. At first I just wanted a little extra to go on vacation. My employer wasn't just going to give me extra time or money, so I decided I had to work another job. If what you want doesn't come to you—you need a way to take it. A part-time job landed in my lap when I met the owner at a happy hour, and as it turned out, they really liked me. They wanted to hire me on fulltime, but since I liked my first employer, I decided to keep both jobs. After some time, I made the money for a vacation.

I started getting offers from practice owners who were trying to expand. Did I want to make some extra money; could I come in and do a few hours at their clinic? I started to realize that if I went to work at a bunch of different clinics doing part time or per diem work, I could make a lot more money than my salary. I wanted to make this happen, so I got down to work. I typed up a letter, and I sent a mass fax out to every clinic in New York City (mind you, this was about fifteen years ago, when faxes were still considered high-tech). To my surprise, my phone started ringing off the hook with people asking when I could work and how high my fees were. I quoted each caller a higher rate than the last, until the fourth or fifth person started to balk. At that point, I knew what the right rate was. So I did the math. I could work fewer hours for a higher salary, or I could work the same job with zero chance of increased pay. And why would I keep working for a fixed salary when I could make more money working less hours at several different practices?

A buddy of mine made a point to me, though. I would be the only one going around to all these places. The only way I could make more money was if I hired more people and gave them a cut. And that was how I started by first staffing company. It worked so well because, in addition to sending my employees, I also went in as an employee so I could talk to the other staffers. I was able to talk up my own company and tell them how great it was. It worked like a charm, and I built up an amazing list of contacts networking this way. That staffing company worked successfully for about two years, at which time I sold it.

Running the staffing company showed me the inner operations and backend business models of a lot of different clinics. I knew how they worked now. I'd had the inside track, and I'd been able to see what they did well and what they did poorly. It had also put me in a position, going from practice to practice, where I already had a bunch of great patients who wanted only to see me. It was clear that the best way to use that to my advantage would be to get all of those patients coming to me, instead of going to them myself.

So I finally made the decision to start my own practice. I went to see all my supposed friends at the various places I'd worked to tell them about it. I told them, "Hey guys, I'm starting my own practice! Don't worry, it's not going to affect your practice. I'm based all the way downtown." To a one, they all turned their backs on me. To them, that was all well and good, but now I was competition. I wasn't really, but they thought of me that way. I was fifty blocks away and there are more than eight million people in New York City! I was furious, but it was eye-opening. This former so-called friends of mine basically blacklisted me. I never forgot that lesson—and I didn't want that to happen to anybody else.

My first year or so I made probably zero money. But by my second year, I had figured a few things out and learned a little more about sales and marketing, so my numbers started to go up. At first told myself I was starting my practice on the side. I started small, but after a year, my accountant came to me and said, "Joe, do you realize that, hour for hour, you made more money working at that practice two days a week for four hours a day, than you did working at the other two jobs full time?"

Now, my accountant had been working for himself for many years. So it was significant when he looked at me and said, "Remember, you will always make more money at your own business than you will working for somebody else." That's something I've always remembered, and that has become one of my main pieces of advice for others.

Of course, I had ups and downs at my practice, and even one really rough patch. But I relied on what I had learned about sales and marketing, and the lessons I want to bring to you. These were all key pieces of knowledge when it came time for my wife to start her practice as well.

My Wife's First Practice
The lessons I learned when I was starting my first practice have never left me. But in life, we not only

have to keep using what we learn, but to keep learning from what we encounter. That's what I try to do when I work with new medpreneurs, and it's what I did almost eight years after starting my own practice when I helped my wife start hers.

My wife and I have two children. She's a pediatric gastroenterologist, and when she was pregnant with our first child she was working for a hospital. She was probably putting in sixty hours a week. And anyone reading this who has children will understand this: during her first trimester, she slept a lot. Basically, if she wasn't at work, she was asleep. I could walk in and out of the house, and she wouldn't wake up. I don't think she knew I was alive for those first three months of her pregnancy. She'd say, "Where are you? I never see you!" And it was because I'd come home, see she was asleep, and go off to the gym. Then I'd come home, see she was sleeping, and get myself something to eat.

The fatigue started to lessen by her second trimester, but her hours got crazier. She was working even more, and we both started to worry about what would happen once our kids were born. When the time approached, the hospital only gave her a brief six weeks of maternity leave (it's a generous eight if you have a C-section). In their opinion it was alright to spend only a total of six weeks with your newborn child before going back to work.

At that point we were both struggling, and we had to try to come up with solutions as far as what to do once she was born: we'd put the baby in daycare; we'd have people watch her; we'd leave her at relatives' houses. We knew we would do whatever we had to do for her. And obviously, it was a lot of stress at the time.

I had my practice, and I was trying to make it grow and generate more money. I felt a lot of pressure to find a way to earn enough money so that my wife could stay home a little bit longer with our baby.

It was amazing that we survived that time after she was born. When we found out that my wife was pregnant with a second child, we both agreed there was no way we could do it again the way we did the first time. I suggested if we cut back, we could live off of one salary, and my wife agreed. After her maternity leave, she would not be going back to work. We started banking her income during the maternity leave in order to practice living on one income.

It was extremely hard. Not only did we have one child in daycare and soon to be starting school, we had the second one coming to take care of. And we didn't know how we could make it work. Then I had an epiphany. I said to her, "You know, if you started your own practice, you could make your own hours." It would still add up to a lot of hours, but I knew it would make a big difference. What we needed then was flexibility. Nobody minds working, and we only expect to be paid for the hours that we work. But that hospital mandated that she work between forty and sixty hours every week. She had to be on call at certain times. And it just wasn't compatible with the main thing she wanted, which was to spend time with our children.

So we decided to start a small practice in one room and see how it would go. No staff, no bells and whistles. We started putting everything in place, and I started working on her website myself, since I knew it would be the main way for people to find her. I set it up with an e-mail capture and appointment-booking program. And as it happened, the website was finished before she even secured a place. It wasn't beautiful; it was just a put-together website, so I could show her how everything would look.

We got our first appointment only about six hours after the website went live. We hadn't listed an address because we didn't even have a location at the time! I couldn't believe it. We were both thinking, "Who is this person?"

At the same time, Google had already cached her website. Even though it was finished, I took it down for about three months. But it was still saved by Google's crawler. And all the while, we knew we had to hurry and find a place for her practice because she already had one patient! So we found a spot. My wife ran her practice there for three months before our second daughter was born. She decided to take some time off after the birth, and during the time off, she found she was taking a lot of phone calls. Hospitals and other physicians were constantly calling to ask when she would be back from maternity leave. We built up such a buzz during her leave that I couldn't believe it— and all because of one website with no marketing.

Because of this one simple thing, people were calling, and we ended up booking them ten to twelve weeks out. When she returned to work, we cleaned out the location and added another room. She was only running her practice one day a week and still making decent money. She was able to do all this and still have most of her time available for the children.

None of her friends could believe it. They all had nannies and had to put their children in programs. Maybe she was only making half of what they made, but she only had to work one day a week. Imagine if she was working five, right? But the way she did it freed up money that would have been spent on a nanny, and freed her up to raise our daughters, take them to sports, Girl Scouts, and other activities, and to be involved in their schooling.

The cash may not equal what her medical school colleagues are making, but her quality of life tends to far surpass theirs. You simply can't put a price on the value of spending the first couple of years with your kids. I work a lot personally, but I've learned to schedule free days when I don't think about work. I spend time with my family, and the reason I have the freedom to do that is because I work for myself.

Coaching

I loved the fact that I was able to help my wife start up a successful practice almost instantaneously, and I hated the feeling I had when I started my own and all my friends who were fellow doctors abandoned me. You could say that the reason I coach and do strategic partnering is that I want people who start their own practices today to have an experience that is more like my wife's and less like mine.

Sometimes students come to my clinic, grab all my brochures, and say "Now I have everything Joe has! I'm going to start my own clinic!" That's fine. Practitioners and healthcare providers can have everything I do, but if they don't know how to implement that, it's useless. It's worth it for some people to hire a coach. If they're losing money anyway, they're in the hole. Even if they pay me 50% of what they have, then what's 50% of nothing? And from my perspective, if I see a business that's losing money and that I know I can turn around to make a profit, why would I not want to? When we implement the strategies that I know work, we consistently turn those failing practices around.

It has also made me a better business person. I learn from my clients' ideas just as they learn from mine. But those ideas have to be tested. Often my clients will have an idea, but not know how to implement it. Or they'll have a concept, but they'll be afraid to take the risk. That's why I'm there. And everyone ends up growing from the experience.

My most recent client, for example, is someone I'm very proud of. He came to me because he was just tired of doing the day-to-day work of his practice. He wanted to be like me and automate so that he was not there as much. We set a goal to achieve this in six months, and we hit that goal. Now he's coming to me saying, "What's the next thing? I have all this free time, and I don't know what to do with myself!" Now that he has automated his practice and freed up time for himself, he has the opportunity to expand or to move in other directions if he wants to. But the first thing I told him to do was take a few days off and celebrate having achieved his goal. It made me feel great, and him too.

I always remember how people treated me when I started, and I would never treat anyone that way. A lot of coaches and consultants out there are trying to make a quick buck. Maybe they used to be practitioners themselves. But if they're not in the trenches of the healthcare world daily, if they don't own their own practice, my faith in them is diminished a little bit.

Some of the skills might be there, but they don't know what's happening up to the present day.

A lot of big companies will come in and just try to sell websites or brochures. They have great sales and marketing, and they know that healthcare practitioners are not always the most business-savvy people out there. But it's not worth it. So my mission is to enlighten private practice owners and to make them more business-savvy. Even if you're not my client, that doesn't mean you should have to fail!

You could say I have a gift for marketing a strategies. Just recently, I sat down in a room with nineteen other private practice owners. I had each of us come up to the mic and give the best marketing strategy we're using right now. No holding back. Soon everybody was competing with the next person to have the best strategy. When we left that day, we each had twenty new strategies to take home. Some of them were simply amazing.

So I sat down and tweaked each and every one. I came up with a new way to try them. My brain is never happier than when working on these, and I'm somebody who loves numbers and statistics. If you show me what you did that worked great for you, and especially if you show me the numbers on it, my favorite thing in the world is to find the one or two things about it we need to change in order to make it extraordinary.

If you want these nineteen strategies, let's schedule a meeting today. Send me an e-mail at privatepracticebusinessacademy@gmail.com.

Nowadays, I still own my own practice, and I still partner with a lot of other practices. So I still have my foot in the door as a practice owner, and I'm still deeply involved with running my own business. But I've discovered that I have a true passion for marketing and sales, and I believe when you have a true passion, you should follow it. That's why I got into the business of consulting and helping other people build a successful practice the way I have many times over.

Chapter Two

Branching Out

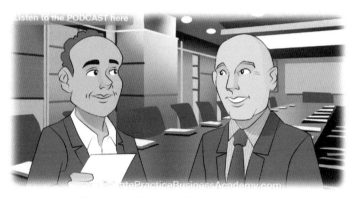

"Do. Or do not. There is no try."

– Yoda, Jedi Master.

Coaching is something a lot of people in the medical community resist, but as you might imagine, I personally think it couldn't be more important. I got into consulting as I did for a reason, and I became a mentor for so many other practitioners. But people resist because they feel that being coached is beneath them or that they should never have to ask anyone for help.

You should. As a rule, if you want to do something well and to be successful at it, you will need someone to teach you.

Finding a Mentor

I myself have mentors whom I still go to. I'm quite proud to admit that. Sometimes people ask me, "How could you coach people if you're being coached yourself?" To me, that question doesn't make sense. I tell them I think I would be doing people a disservice if I only gave them one point of view. Having been coached myself by so many different people, I feel like I've heard from sources with every different perspective imaginable.

Being a great practitioner doesn't necessarily make you a great businessperson. That's why I spend so much time being formally coached, as well as just picking the brains of my colleagues and asking for their ideas. It's also why I like to share my ideas with my own coaching clients, and in return mastermind with my own clients as well. There is a saying that your mentors are the five people you spend the most time with—and I try to spend time with people who will inspire me to be as successful and creative as possible.

If I'd had a mentor all those years ago when I started my first practice, it would have sped up my learning curve dramatically. I wouldn't have made all those mistakes. Now, don't get me wrong. Those mistakes were essential for my learning curve. They helped, but they were very costly as well. But when I go to a practice owner now and tell them what steps we have to take to avoid those pitfalls, it's amazing how fast we can leapfrog the cash flow struggles I had back then. I was just able to partner with another practice owner in

New Jersey, and we went from zero to $100,000 over only nine months because I was able to apply the experience I had through the strategies we implemented.

They are simply things that a new business owner wouldn't do. If you have a partnership in which one person provides the "sweat equity" and the other is responsible for the "brain equity," I think it's a win-win scenario.

I have success stories of practice owners who went from -$50,000 to +$5,000 monthly in about forty days, because I was able to look at their practice with a new set of eyes. That helped us to cut their costs and eliminate their practices' weaknesses.

A good mentor, such as myself, can come into a situation, analyze it dispassionately, and tweak it to make it succeed. However, A mentor doesn't always have to come from outside, like me, and look at your entire practice. Mentoring can be a philosophy and a system you can implement within your practice and truly help it grow from the inside. Recently, I worked with a new private practice owner, and we started a joint mentoring program for the practice's marketing liaison. In very little time, the clinic's morale and numbers skyrocketed. Not to mention the fact that the owner is now much less skeptical of the marketing results. The power of mentoring is something never to lose sight of.

Making the Jump

Starting your own practice is a big step. It doesn't need to be a big office, or be open multiple days a week, or even take you away from your day job, but it's still a significant undertaking. And to be honest, my observation is that people usually make that decision when they're disgruntled. It's very rarely about money. What it is about, is having that freedom to do what you want.

For the young Joe Simon, it was about affording a vacation. For my wife, it was having time to spend with our young daughters. I'm sure you can think of something you would do with some extra time and money if you didn't have to work forty or sixty hours a week. Few people just care about money in and of itself. They care about what they can do with it. And freedom is truly the reason most people make the jump into becoming the owners of their own private practices.

Finding Your Way

When I meet with a consulting client, the first thing I do is sit down with them and try to break down their practice. We go through everything they do. And we don't just look at their business; we look at their life. Why? Everyone who is running a business is doing so with a goal in mind, and the only way to make your practice work the way you want it to is to go in knowing what you want out of it.

In the end, certain things are true of almost every practice owner—whether you're a dentist, acupuncturist, chiropractor, physical therapist, or whatever you may be. You want freedom. You want independence. The reason you've built up a private practice or are trying to start one is so that you can leverage the people who are working for you.

I use that first conversation we have to try to find out what they need most, and in that discussion, I always try to come up with one idea for how to get rid of that problem, or "pain point" as I call it. It may not be the final answer, but it's something we can take and say, "Let's try this first."

Do some of these most common pain points that I encounter sound familiar to you?

Family in distress - Sometimes the pain point is that their marriage is on the rocks because they have no time for it. Maybe they're never home, or never get to see their kids. To be honest, that's what I hear about the most. And it breaks my heart when I think of my two little girls at home, five and two years old.

Financial Struggles - Other people are about to go bankrupt because a hospital just bought out the doctor referral group from which they were getting all their referrals. Now they have no idea where to get referrals from, or how to keep their practices open.

Unhelpful Staff - In many practices, the staff is not on board with the company's vision, which in the end is simply destroying the practitioner's dream of independence.

Insurance/Billing Issues - Often, a practice can't stay in the black simply because insurance companies aren't paying or due to other billing-related issues.

If you recognize yourself or your own pain points in any of the people I've been describing, I want you to keep reading. Because that means you're just the kind of practitioner my coaching and experience is built around.

When the people I meet with realize that they can free themselves for their families or keep their businesses open by making six or seven big but simple changes, they tend to be ready to implement those business strategies right away. I know from my one or two clients on the West Coast of Canada, they're much more accepting of my method up there, which is very cash-based and cash-driven. In the United States, it's hard to break the mentality that asks the question, "Why should I invest in the education and marketing I need to get people to come in off the street and pay me cash, when I could just get my insurance payment instead?"

But it's becoming more common. The United States is moving more towards cash-based practices. If you find yourself still struggling with that question, think about your own pain points, and think about how you want to change them. That's what I want to help you do.

The Day Job and the Fear of Failing

If you have a day job going while you start off, that's perfectly fine. I recommend you keep yours for the time being. In fact, if you can funnel money from the day job into your new practice, I think that's a great way to help yourself out.

There's never any shame in working a day job while running a practice. One fellow physical therapist I know started a cash-based practice, brought it to a successful position, and then put it on hold when she went through a divorce. She knew it was easier to get insurance and a mortgage with a non-fluctuating paycheck. But once she had that in order, she went back to working for herself and made her practice more successful than ever. There's nothing the matter with that—it just means she's proven twice how successful the business model can be.

There's no minimum requirement for what percentage of your working life your practice has to take up before you're a private practice owner. As soon as you see that first patient, you're a business owner—and you can do whatever you want with that business. I remember when I first started, my office was only open Tuesday and Thursday evenings from four o'clock to seven o'clock. Pretty transparently the hours of somebody keeping his day job, but it was enough to start. Those three hours twice a week built up and paid off.

Absolutely everyone starts out with a certain fear. I know you're thinking *'What if I fail?'* I thought that too. It's a normal fear to have. Frankly, I want you to fail, and fail fast. When I say I want you to fail, maybe I should put it another way: I *know* you will fail. But you'll only fail temporarily, and when you fail, I want you to say, "Okay, I made a mistake. Let's figure out what went wrong, fix it, and move on. You're going to lose some battles, but you'll win the war. And you'll still have that day job to fall back on for safety, just in case.

A mentor that I've since had once told me, "Fail fast. Failure isn't failure; it's just testing. That's what marketers call failing." I told him I was a healthcare practitioner, not a marketer. But he just told me, "Joe, everyone's a marketer!" It's all true, and it's some of the best advice I've ever been given. Sometimes I wish that as Future Joe I could go back in time, meet my previous self, and tell Past Joe exactly what to do. But I didn't have that, and that's why I'm sharing all of this with you. As I always tell people when they're afraid of making mistakes, the worst thing that could happen is that you just don't get paid. And this book is about making sure that doesn't happen to you.

Cutting the Cord

As you probably know, a lot of healthcare professionals today are working for hospitals or hospital-based practices. Others are working for other doctors in private practices. They might be making decent money, but they're often not making what they'd like to or what they feel they're truly worth. If you're reading this book and don't already have your own practice, there's a decent chance you're one of these people. You're interested in being your own boss and making your own money, but you're still on the fence for one reason or another.

One thing I want to do with this book is to show you that branching out on your own as a cash-based practice is something you can do, and I have a lot of advice for you when you do it. Remember that if an insurance company only wants to pay you a $20 copay, they're essentially saying that your value is $20 in that situation. When a patient pays you a $20 copay from their pocket, they immediately equate that amount to your value.

I think—and I suspect you think too—that your value is much more than that. And in your own practice, you can set your own value. If you are overvalued, the market will tell you. If you are undervalued, that's something most practitioners don't realize—and sometimes they need someone to tell them.

One thing that I tell a lot of people I work with and that has become a sort of mantra for me is that we need to stop complaining about the state of healthcare and start making a difference. We need to stop talking about problems and start figuring out ways to solve them. The strongest way to take matters into your own hands is to start your own medical practice rather than remain part of somebody else's.

Case Study: Dr. Lisa Holland

I got some great insights on the process of "cutting the cord" from a previous medical employer when I spoke with Dr. Lisa Holland, a doctor of physical therapy who cut the cord from her hospital practice and now runs her own cash-based yoga therapy studio. Lisa had been practicing for over ten years when she did it, and by the time she went fully out on her own in 2011, she had found an area of specialization outside of general physical therapy that really spoke to her abilities and resonated with her patients.

Lisa discovered Yoga when recovering from her own pregnancy, and eventually she became convinced that lifestyle-type care was the wisest way to go in terms of how to treat people with chronic pain or disabilities. In 2005, Lisa tried opening a private boutique-style studio while continuing her day job, but found that trying to manage two huge elements of her professional life at once wasn't successful.

But as more and more people showed interested in being her private clients, she realized that if given her full attention and treated as a genuine business, her side venture could be very successful. As she put it to me, "Around 2011, I just realized that I really, really thought my model of care delivery was a better way to go for getting people better, faster. I run cash based, so there wasn't the whole headache. A lot of my work in the hospital, and even in the clinics, was so much of the stress and tiredness of just keeping up the dynamics of insurance mandated care, as opposed to what I could really do, and do this more efficiently. So in 2011, I just said, let's make this full time. This is no longer my hobby. This is my practice."

That was a bold move on Lisa's part, and it's been a very successful one for her. She now gets 95% of her clients from marketing and word of mouth rather than physician referrals, and that's a very good place to be in. As she explained to me, "What's important is that entrepreneurial spirit. If there's a yearning for you, and a confidence in yourself and your abilities, that's the utmost need. No matter what, you still need to be willing to work hard. But when you're working on your own, it's a different kind of hard. There's a little bit more of a gratification, because it is whatever you're producing, you feel like it's of you."

That's been true for me, and I know it will be true for you as well. When you're working for yourself, you're the only one who puts a value on your time, so it becomes that much more rewarding—both figuratively and financially. So what steps do you need to take if you want to achieve that? That's what I hope to share with you. Keep reading, and if you want to catch up with more information about Lisa and her practice, check out my interview with her at http://privatepracticebusinessacademy.com/cut-cord-belly-guru-llc-founder-dr-lisa-holland/.

You'll notice that one thing Lisa didn't immediately do from the start, and that was quit her day job. She built her practice up, and when it was able to sustain itself, then she cut the cord.

Outfitting your Space Digitally

Once acquired, your office space is going to need to be set up for your practice, and ideally in the most effective way possible. In that regard, you can set up your software and technology to make things far easier than they would have been several years ago. Ten years has made a big difference in what it costs to set up a practice, and another ten will make an even bigger one. Many practices—startups especially among them—work much better today because they can be so virtual.

Phone and Answering Services:

Needless to say, a phone line is necessary. But the traditional way to get that has changed. You don't need to call AT&T or Verizon and get a line drilled in and installed in your office anymore. Google Voice works great, saves money, and is easier to install. Some resources I like include a web service called ringcentral.com, or another called evoice.com. Essentially, these allow you to set up a separate line with a voicemail system, but it causes the call to ring through to your cell phone. That way, it seems like you have a staffed, full-service professional practice, but in reality you get the call on your own private cell phone.

You can let it ring and screen the call by letting it go to voicemail, or answer if you have the time. If you want a real human answering the phone for you, but aren't in position yet to hire a secretary, there are answering services you can hire. Of course, that's another cost. So if you're just starting out, I'd recommend sticking with a service such as Ringcentral or eVoice.

If you only have one or two people calling you each week, in no way do you need an answering service. Answer your own phone; let it go to voice mail, or have some way to capture the number so you can call it back. The exception, of course, would be if you have the kind of practice where you need to respond immediately to someone's emergency call, in which case, you might want to invest in an answering service earlier.

Start off with a Website:

A very early step you should take when starting a practice might seem obvious in today's world, but it's one that people do sometimes leave out. You need your own website. I meet with a lot of doctors who want to leave this out, because they think they'll have to spend thousands on it. You don't. What you need is simplicity and presence. Sure there are unsavory characters out there who will charge you thousands of dollars or whatever you're willing to pay, but that kind of person is called a con artist.

Scheduling Software:

Finally, you're going to need to set your practice up with a scheduling software of some sort. Obviously, if you have patients, you need to keep track of when they are coming in. You shouldn't just be writing it down on a piece of paper in this day and age. Of course, you know that in the medical world everyone is very tied into Electronic Medical Records and making sure they are linked with scheduling software, but in the beginning, you can still keep things very simple. You want to keep track of when each patient is coming in. You want to be alerted of when they're coming, and you want the same system to alert the patient (or failing that, you want to make sure to give them a follow-up call).

As long as a system is doing that for you, it's actually doing what you need. Google Calendar is something I've used, and I'd still be alright with using it professionally even today. I use it to keep my personal online appointment book, and it works fantastically. It has that feature where it reminds the client for an upcoming appointment—which is labor-saving for you—so I think it's a great, cost effective tool for people just starting out.

The key mentality is to look at everything you do, and think, "How can this help my practice? How can this grow my reputation and my business?" With that attitude constantly in mind, you're going to find success, and the strategies I lay out here will open up to you.

With my consulting clients, I'm always checking in after some period of time, seeing how progress is going, and driving my messages into them one-on-one. I'm there to tell them, "Alright, we really need to get this going," and keep their noses to the grindstone. I wish I could do that with my readers, but I know from experience that if you absorb the lessons here, you will be able to turn yourself into the successful practitioner you want to be within a matter of months.

That's why hiring a coach can be such a groundbreaking step for any practice. Whether a clinic is a success really has almost nothing to do with assets, premises, or qualifications. It has to do with the mindset of the people there. I can't count how many times I've seen a small shift in attitude cause a seismic shift in fortunes. As the practitioner, you have to be a leader in mindset and attitude. And if you still have the old attitude of waiting for patients to show up at your door and letting things happen for you instead of making them happen yourself, you're going to need to make some changes.

Chapter Three

Finding Your Place in the World

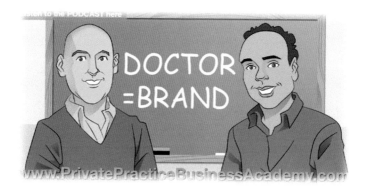

"A person who never made a mistake never tried

anything new."

– *Albert Einstein, physicist.*

I'm a big promoter of niche practices, and I'll say right from the start: If you're not niching down your practice, you certainly should be. If you're good at one thing, that's your niche, and that will be the reason people pay you for that exact specialty.

The niche is something that comes up very often in my conversations with new clients; people have a hard time figuring out what makes them unique. When I ask people, sometimes I get a cookie-cutter answer that isn't much use, and we have to delve a little deeper in order to find a substantial answer to the question of what sets them apart.

Maybe you're familiar with the fact that when orthopedic specialists perform surgery, they have what we call in daily parlance "the hand guy" or "The wrist guy" or "the knee guy." It means they know their own areas thoroughly, and they're always in demand for their particular niches. People in other disciplines tend to neglect to do this, to their detriment. I've found that niching down too deep is really impossible. The more specific the service you offer, the more you will attract people who need that service and are willing to pay for an expert in it.

The tough part is, though, most people simply don't know what their niche is. They want to start something new, break out on their own, and do their own thing, but they don't know exactly how. And that's the real challenge.

For years, I thought I understood niching down, but I really didn't. I'd heard other people talking about it, but in the back of my mind, I still thought it was slightly nuts to say, "I treat head and neck injuries only." I was the first person to argue against niching down. It seemed so dumb; why would I want to lose all the other patients?

It didn't hit me until I started partnering with other physical therapists and opening up practices. I once partnered with a friend to start a practice, and I took the task of writing our promotion materials and website copy. But when I did it, I was writing everything as if I were running the clinic. The people who were coming in were basically patients for me—but I was never there. The therapists who worked there kept getting patients with types of injuries they didn't treat. So I wanted to address the problem. I asked the staff what they did treat, and it turned out to be injuries that would be encountered by high school athletes.

So I went back to the drawing board. I rewrote the site, and I called a staff meeting. I told everyone, "Guys, from now on, we only treat high school athletes. If someone out of school comes in with neck pain we say, 'I'm sorry, but right now, we're focusing on high school athletes; that's all we treat.'" Even my business partner thought I was crazy when I said this. In his mind, we were giving money away when we turned away patients that way. But I asked him to give me one month just to see how it worked.

That one month changed everybody's mind. Our numbers quadrupled in the span of thirty days—just because we changed and narrowed our message down from, "We do everything," to, "We only treat high school athletes." Sure, other practices in the area would take high school athletes, but why would you go to them when you could go to the clinic that specializes? We even told the other clinics in the area, "We'll send you everyone else; give us your high school athletes!" Of course, some of those other practices were friendly about it, and some weren't. And I can tell you which ones we sent our other patients to. That's good business.

Now, we have a great relationship with two other physical therapy practices in the area. It's rare that you can say physical therapy practices work together, because they usually look at each other as competition. But if you're niched down the way you should be, you don't have to occupy the same profession, and you could physically occupy the same location.

So that ended up being a perfect niche. Besides which, it's fun working with kids. They also recover faster, which makes us feel good, besides making them feel good. Monetarily, it's a dream because people are willing to spend any amount of money on their kids. The backend secret is now parents are coming to us with their problems, and there's no harm in taking that business if the family is already a client of yours.

The experience I had with that practice was a great lesson for me. Living that and going through that experience has changed the way I work with my clients; it has changed the way I partner with people, and has even changed the way I run my own practices. Why say you do everything when you can say you do something you like to do? It's amazing when that happens: everyone's happy and you make more money.

Finding Your Own Profitable Niche

I'll give away the secret right here: nobody knows what niche works right off the bat. Even I didn't know. I've made mistakes, thinking one thing is going to be a homerun or is a sure-fire solution and finding that it doesn't work. It can be difficult to admit you don't know something, especially as a qualified practitioner. But there can be a lot of power in it as well. Once you've admitted you don't have your niche, the vista of opportunities opens up to you. Sometimes you just have to go through that process.

The idea that I'm giving you about picking a niche isn't a new one. It's one I heard time and time again when I was first starting out and going to a lot of conferences and speakers' events. And every time, the speakers I heard would try to give some formula for how to pick a correct niche. Their problem was that they missed the most basic problem: sometimes you just don't know. In a recent closed-door meeting with forty practice owners, we strategized on possible profitable niches they could pursue immediately.

It might take you some time, and that's alright. You didn't have the benefit of being in a room with me and thirty-nine others to work on your niche with you. You might have to see everyone at first in order to realize what you attract in terms of clientele.

Give yourself those first six months that I mentioned in chapter one. Test out everything. All you want to do is see what works. Especially if you're a small practice that's just starting out, maneuverability is your greatest asset. You're going to see who you attract, and what kind of patient feels the strongest connection with you. The formula for attraction is notoriously elusive, but once you start to understand how it's operating, you can harness its power for your practice. Personally, I make year-long strategic business plans for my own practice—and I know what huge changes can take place by the six month mark.

If your niche is that you treat pregnant women, it might not work as well for you if you're a man as it would if for a woman who has already had a child, because clients could feel a female would better relate to them. That has nothing to do with how good you are as a practitioner. Your real life attempts to find a niche will have very many more factors at play. It's just a small example, but it can be helpful to keep in mind.

There are more niches out there than you might imagine. I know a therapist who is building a huge practice around the niche of treating athletes who do parkour, a sport related to gymnastic stunts on city geography. It's a sport a lot of people don't even know exists, but it has a hugely dedicated following who have specialized health problems, and who go directly to him when they need help.

When you're first starting, I say to throw everything against the wall and see what sticks. I know it feels like the worst method, but after six months, you're really going to start to see what's coming down off the wall and what's staying. Then if you really dig down and hone in on that, you can build everything else around it. It might take six months. It might take a year. But if it takes more than that, you're really not paying attention.

A great example I can give is of a certain women's health group in North Carolina. The practitioner essentially targets only pregnant and postpartum women. You might think there's not enough in it, but she's a huge success. In one of our clinics we specialize in facial paralysis. It's actually hard to make your niche too small. There will always be enough people who have the problem you address, and you want them going directly to you.

I even know one doctor who was so inventive in finding his niche, that in the process he essentially created a new kind of practice. Dr. Alejandro Badilla, an orthopedic hand surgeon, started what is now known as an orthopedic urgent care clinic. He's branded it as

OrthoNow and expanded it. It's a specialized orthopedic practice, but it homes in on treating patients who otherwise would end up going to an emergency room, waiting, being charged an arm and a leg, and eventually getting referred to someone like Alejandro anyway. It means faster, better care for the injured person, and a lot of business for Alejandro—and I think it's an amazing model. Patients will drive forty-five minutes because it saves them six hours in the emergency room. Sometimes finding your niche means creating it yourself.

Your niche is personal; it relates not just to what will make you the most money, but to what you're best at, and what you like to do. Combine that with something in demand, and you have it made—but of course, it's not always that simple. I can't tell you in just a few lines how to find your niche, because it's such an individual and really unquantifiable process. I'm confident that by the end of this book, have a better understanding of how you can really carve out your own personalized niche.

For now, let's take a look at the example of one professional whose niche wasn't working for him.

Case Study: Dr. William Bennett (AKA my friend Bill)

One of my clients, Bill, is two months into his own practice as a concierge physical therapist—so well before his six test months would be up. He started off with patients from his former position. Now, I'm not a proponent of taking clients from your former employer, but according to him, these people decided to follow him on their own. And business started off doing well.

However, the clients were being discharged because, well . . . they were getting better. He kept some for a health and wellness program, but on the whole, they were riding off into the sunset. So at this point—inevitably, if somewhat delayed—he finally faced the challenge of finding new clients. He now realized he was at a disadvantage because he'd personally been going to the clients rather than having them come to him—and, of course, he was losing time that way. So he came to me. I told him concierge therapist could be a great niche, but you have to look at the downside of it as well.

A number of factors made it a difficult niche to leverage for a profit. It's a one man show, which means you can't hire anyone on to expand the business of the practice. Traveling everywhere raises travel expenses, and costs you a lot of money simply in the amount of time that you spend getting from one client to another. Where would he get new patients? His old method, along with many of his clients, had come from his old employer. And what's more, he brought me another problem that was holding his practice back: "It seems like I spend most of my day on the phone with insurance companies. I can't leverage my time. I can't do any marketing. I can't do anything!"

By this time, he had a lot of pain points in his operation, and he didn't even know if he was on the right track at all. The only thing he did know was that the money per client was far better than when he was working for somebody else. Seeing only two people a day, he was earning more money than he did working an eight-hour shift—and he wanted to keep his practice going so he could continue that situation.

As I pointed out to him, that little calculation he did meant freedom. Being one of the new medprenuers meant that the equivalent of an eight-hour shift was done after two hours, and that meant more time for him and what he wanted to do. If Bill wanted to take off in the middle of the day and hang out with me or get coffee, there was nothing to stop him. That's a great feeling. And that great feeling can be even greater if we can get past pain points like Bill's—not being able to leverage time spent with insurance firms, not being able to leverage marketing time, and, hugely, not having a set location.

So what did I tell him? Bearing in mind he had a great start and was making a name for himself, I said, "Let's take a look at all the places where your clients are right now. Is there a central location you're going to, or are you scattered?"

He was a little bit scattered, but overall, 90% of his clients were in one certain neighborhood. So I said, "OK. Let's see if we can team up with another healthcare professional in that neighborhood. During this time that you've recently freed up for yourself, let's find a health professional that will sub-lease you space—maybe one or two days a week, even, just to keep your expenses low and to test the waters." Most health care providers will be happy to rent space since, of course, they're looking to make money from their offices when they have dead time.

Sub-Leasing and Finding a Space

Sub-leasing turned out to be a great solution for Bill, and that's no surprise. It's an ideal solution for a huge number of people who are just starting their own practices. You don't have to pay for electricity, and you don't have to pay for furniture. I'd say it's the best way to go if you're an absolute beginner. It was certainly step one for me when I was starting, and I don't regret it. As I mentioned, I didn't quit my day job to start with, but what I did do was find a place. And that'll be the number one thing for you as well. You simply need somewhere to work out of.

At the time, I absolutely couldn't afford leasing my own space, but I could afford sub-leasing. So I reached out to virtually every physician I knew and brought up the subject. Of course, people are going to be eager to capitalize on those times when they aren't using a space that they're already paying for, even if it's only one or two days a week. It's not something you need to be reticent about, because if you ask doctors if you can sub-lease their space, they will almost all respond with open arms. You're basically offering to give them money, after all, and using up the time when the space would be empty.

Sometimes you can even hire the staff that's already there to do some side work for you. I couldn't, but that didn't stop me—and it shouldn't stop you either. These days, I'm sure you could rent a whole office for less than I would have had to pay back then, but sub-leasing is still really the way to go.

If you absolutely can't sub-lease, look into renting out a similar place at a day-rate for a while. Almost any healthcare practitioner could easily do that for what they would get in reimbursement, even if it was private-pay or insurance based. You'd basically only need to see one patient a day to cover expenses, and that's a home run. Plus, with the networking that's involved in a place like that, you would meet a large number of people who could help you grow your practice later on.

The third possibility, which is one that I didn't even think of when I started my practice, is to go to your patients instead of asking them to come to you. It might conjure up images of the old country doctor making house calls with his little black bags, but the concierge practice, as it is called, is a legitimate option, and it's one that I've taken advantage of as well. I've shown up at people's houses and helped them out using whatever I had on hand at the time.

If you're absolutely dead set against sub-leasing space or renting an office, being a concierge practitioner is an option. It is important to remember the travel will cost you money and valuable time, but it can be made to work. If the money is there, and somebody says, "I'll pay you to come to my house because I'm unable or don't have the time to leave," then that's certainly something to consider. But remember what your ultimate goal is. And a concierge practice is hard to scale and sell someday.

But any way you do it, the most important point is that you need a home base. Even if you have a concierge practice, you want to avoid the image of the unprofessional, itinerant, travelling-salesman doctor. At some point, if you're successful enough for long enough in your practice, you're going to consider going street level with it. It could be in the middle of the country, or it could be in a big city like New York or

Miami. Going street level, like any large step, has significant potential risks and rewards.

It's very expensive, but obviously, very visible to new clients. It's fair to say that it will guarantee you a certain number of new clients from walk-ins per week, depending on location. But the decision has to be made on the basis of whether that will outstrip your expected expense.

Telemedicine and the Global Practice

One thing to remember when finding a location for your practice is depending on your specialty, you may in some cases be able to leap over the question of location altogether—both yours and that of your client.

I spoke not long ago with Jessica Drummond, the CEO of the Integrative Pelvic Health Institute, who explained how she also does private nutritional consulting for clients all over the globe: "I do it either over the phone or on Skype. I have about ten to fifteen private patients I work with really in depth, getting to the root cause of their issues, and doing a lot of coaching. One thing about nutrition is that you can give a person a list of foods they should eat based on their food sensitivity results and hormone testing, but food is such an emotional thing that there's a lot of coaching that goes along with actually implementing those changes over the long term. So I do a lot of long distance coaching with my private patients, and I can help keep them on track, even if they're all the way in Singapore."

It's obviously not a replacement for your physical office, but if you have a specialty or service that allows you to consult over long distances using the telephone or VOIP and web-conferencing services such as Skype, there's another great potential income stream for you, with very little overhead.

New developments have arisen in the world of telemedicine, and they're developments that you could profitably take advantage of for your business. My own state of New York is one of several where a new state law allows practitioners to bill insurance for telemedicine. Previously, the prevailing concept was that if you could treat someone over the phone or over Skype, you could charge a fee—but you couldn't bill the insurance companies. The companies simply didn't recognize telephone or Skype consultations as legitimate treatment.

This new law is going to bring a lot of changes to how people are currently practicing—or to how they should be. For instance, I was recently approached by a large firm interested in setting up a broad network of physicians. Now, it had previously been fairly difficult for a physician to team up with other practitioners, be they other physicians, physical therapists, chiropractors, or what have you. State laws got in the way; they may not have been close by, and the whole concept of entrepreneurship was different in many people's minds.

But now a platform is being set up that can really connect physicians and other practitioners within a group—without physical distance as an impediment—and let them really get the patient everything he or she needs. Let's say a woman comes into a practice to see a physical therapist. That physical therapist might very well be able to tell her, "Here's how I can treat you. And here's something else I noticed that you'd need to see another specialist for."

But how often does that happen? For so long, a practitioner's greatest fear was that if they referred a patient to another practitioner, the patient wouldn't come back, and they would lose the money they otherwise had coming to them. This telemedicine network will allow you to call another doctor through Skype, consult on what's needed, and bill that to insurance without a risk of losing the patient. It helps both medical professionals, and it helps the patient. Your client never leaves your office, and you get the extra information you need immediately from an expert who gets to charge for it. And of course, the patient doesn't have to wait weeks for another appointment.

The first provider gets the opportunity to look like a superhero, because they can demonstrate the huge network of people they can reach out to at a moment's notice based on what they see the patient may need. A primary care physician could call a specialist, or vice versa. This is a breakthrough concept, and I feel telemedicine will really take off with this. New York, California, Georgia, and Texas have laws that allow this already, and I feel that the tide is turning towards it. If you're not sure about where you practice, do a Google search and see what the law is in your state.

I tried telemedicine before. In the past, my practice had an e-commerce platform set up where patients could log in and ask for advice. We tested the platform in beta about a year ago—and it didn't work. For whatever reason, there just wasn't enough traffic. In my view, it's because the trust simply wasn't there.

People didn't know how this was going to help them or why they were paying a fee.

Personally, I think the partner I had on the product pulled it too early. There were plenty of things that could have been tweaked—from the price point to the title to the landing page—to try to get a better result. I always encourage testing your marketing, but that's just what we didn't get to do with my version of telemedicine.

Now, what I'm really looking forward to is trying out the possibilities of Skype-enabled, networked, provider-billed telemedicine. It think it will really change how we all practice.

Corporate Practice and Beyond

Of course, the options I have been discussing are not the only ways in which you can find a place to start your entrepreneurial practice. A lot of professionals have approached me in the past with a question about how to start their own practice within a corporate office. That's a natural idea to think of. It means you're going directly to where there's a lot of money, which, if you play your cards right, can be spent on your practice's service.

I want to give you the example of a friend and colleague of mine, Dr. Kelly Lease, who runs Kelly Lease physical therapy. One of the things that I admire strongly about Kelly is that she's a strongly driven person who goes directly to what she wants. And what she wanted, originally was to be a dancer. She went for it all the way, designed her life around being physically fit and active—and dancing.

But when she was seventeen, she injured her ankle and was told she would never dance again. As I hope you haven't had the chance to find out for yourself, it's very tough to have dreams crushed at such a young age. But when she received physical therapy for her injury, it made such a difference for her that she actually was able to return to competitive dancing again, and then to teach dancing.

But the gift that physical therapy gave her, as well as the knowledge she acquired of flexibility and the human body, encouraged her to want to make that positive difference for other people's mobility and to become a physical therapist herself. I think it's wonderful that she found that pathway from a personal disappointment to a great career as a physical therapist. I've found that a lot of people in our profession have a pretty inspiring background story about how they got into physical therapy.

The best news is that Kelly is still involved in dance. And her whole story makes her a great example of what I've already written about here—finding your niche. Kelly was someone whose niche was essentially with her first, and then her practice came later. Her deep firsthand knowledge of the challenges faced by dancers who require physical therapy gave her very attractive qualifications as a professional right from the start. And her success in that field today is a great example of how one little step can change a whole career.

Kelly's ability to specialize within a niche eventually landed her a job as the staff physical therapist for Broadway's famously intensive, dance-heavy production of *The Lion King* and led her to the attention of a company called Plus One, which basically has a lock on the practices within America's biggest corporate and financial offices. Plus One led her to the position of running the physical therapy practice within Goldman Sachs' New Jersey office.

Kelly found that working within a corporation can provide a boost and a base without preventing an entrepreneurially-minded person from growing their practice. As she told me, "It got to the point where people would tell me all the time, 'I don't know what you're doing, but keep doing it, because patients are pouring in. Everyone's thrilled. People are happy.'"

Kelly also explained to me how she found that running a practice within a corporate context can be very rewarding, but also require a deft touch, saying, "It was a great experience there, and it was a slightly different type of model than a practice on the street because I was dealing with a very specialized patient population. People are very intelligent. They're very motivated to get better. And, frankly, you're basically in people's houses—you're right in the middle of the corporate culture. Of course, you always want to please the client and have the highest satisfaction rate available. But it's even more of a delicate balance when your office is located within their headquarters. There's pluses and minuses to both."

Through her experience at Goldman Sachs, Kelly had success working at Johnson and Johnson as well. There she ran a practice within the company as basically a fees service—a completely cash-based practice within a corporate context. At this point, you may be thinking, "Sure. But how can I get involved in this part of the industry from where I stand now?" Not everyone will follow Kelly's exact path, and most people trying to get involved in corporate practice will be coming to the company itself.

Obviously, if a company has a health center, as many large companies do, they have a built-in contact point. In the past, that was my method of approach. Essentially, I would go to the company's health center and explain my services. I was offering value, in other words. Of course, at that time, when I was approaching firms, I wouldn't go on about the value I would bring in to my own practice. My emphasis was on the value I could bring to their patients. Obviously, the value I wanted to bring attention to was time management, which as you'll see as we go on, is an essential skill for any practitioner in the first place. That was their main concern because they wanted to keep their healthcare costs down, and having excellent time management is the only way to do that without sacrificing quality.

These are still the key points to hit when approaching firms. And it's equally important to remember that one big thing that applies everywhere in the world of business: don't be afraid to use your connections. Never burn bridges, because you may need them to get you past something later. Even a private patient you've had may belong to a corporate organization that you need to connect with.

So there's no one single way to get a position as a corporate practitioner, but the key element is getting your foot through that crack in the door. You can do that through a company like Plus One or through networking, or you can simple do it by getting on the horn and showing them what you can bring.

Kelly, too, eventually reached the point you have reached if you are reading this book seriously. She wanted to start her own private practice. In her own words: "Patients just kept flooding in to come see me. Physical therapy was really in such high demand. Year after year, the numbers would just spike, and the biggest referral was really by word of mouth. It was almost like we didn't even have to advertise the physical therapy, because if we did, I'd be there Twenty-four/seven. There wasn't enough time in the day.

"So I started to feel like definitely people were noticing that I was in demand there, and I was working hard and willing to do whatever it took to get people in, give them the quality of care. But I started to think not that I was unhappy, but that I should just have my own practice, because I'm basically running the show anyway.

"I really was at almost a breaking point, where I said, I love what I do; I like these patients. I like this company, and they like me. It's a win/win for both of us. We just had this third party involved that we don't really need to deal with. I can easily just do this on my own."

I think Kelly's a great example for all of us, whether we're interested in a corporate practice or not. She found a perfect niche for her skills and experience, made it work for her, grew a successful practice, and knew when to branch out on her own to a completely private business. The strategies and principles that worked for her were the same ones that you'll need in your own practice.

Chapter Four

Know Your Tribe and Speak Their Language

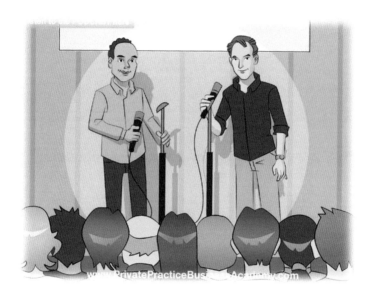

The media wants overnight successes (so they have someone to tear down). Ignore them. Ignore the early adopter critics that never have enough to play with. Ignore your investors that want proven tactics and predictable instant results. Listen instead to your real customers, to your vision and make something for the long haul. Because that's how long it's going to take,

guys.

– Seth Godin

I like to refer to a practice's patient population as a "tribe," because like a tribe they're a group of individuals who are tightly bound together and immediately identifiable by commonalities. So what's the theme of your tribe? It should be something that defines your practice still further—that's how narrowed down I want to get.

Six months or a year into your practice, you're established with the space, staff, website, systems and other elements you need to have in place. But if you haven't settled on a niche market that works for you and can bring in clientele, now is the time to take advantage of that opportunity. You've had months to gather data, and this is where your tracking, your analytics, and even your office staff come into play in helping you arrange and analyze information.

This doesn't just apply to new practices. Established practitioners may not have the flexibility in their business to do what I suggested a new business owner do, and try out lots of niches. In this situation, too, the best way to go is to use demographics to home in on that niche. An established practice will have an even greater body of data with which to work.

Demographics

When you first start out, you probably feel like all you want is patients. You want them to come through your door, and you want them to pay you for what you do. You certainly need that, but probably just as important, or more, is their demographic information, especially at this stage of the game.

A person might come for three visits, feel better, and leave. You may say to yourself "Why didn't they stay for twelve session?" or "Why did that patient never refer anybody?" If a patient referred a lot of people, it's equally important for you to know that. Of course, the answer to these questions lies only in that client's brain, but we can get very useful data-based answers to this questions using demographics, and those answers can help you grow your practice.

You want to know what neighborhood people are from, how old they are, whether they are male or female, what they do for a living, their marital status, whether they have a family. All these things are hugely important because they help you know who is coming to you, and therefore who you can target.

If you use this data correctly, you can make your niche incredibly specific. If you start seeing a lot of female soccer players, you can start to say you specialize in female soccer players. Or high school and college level girls' soccer. You might be surprised, but when you start getting those girls' soccer players in, pretty soon you'll be getting the whole family jumping in. A lot of average people have the mentality that if they're already at the doctor, they might as well come in for whatever malady they might have. And there's more business.

I know practitioners who have specialized even further and billed themselves as experts not just on, say, high school and college level girls' soccer plays, but on one particular injury that they're prone to—and knowing your data is the only way to isolate that. Paying attention to your demographics and really knowing your numbers is probably the best resource you can create for yourself. Running a patient analysis—studying client demographics—is one of the first things I do these days when I come into a practice to consult, and sometimes I don't even charge for it if we're just meeting for the first time.

I just consulted with a physical therapist in New York City who was targeting professional clients with pelvic health issues. Since she was on Electronic Medical Records, I could immediately pull up her client data and ask why she had so many Medicare clients. That segment made up over 30% of her clientele. She said, "I guess they've been coming to me for so long that they don't want to see someone else." It didn't occur to her that she could leave that lower-revenue segment behind and concentrate on what she was trying to grow. This client was focusing on being a pelvic floor rehabilitation specialist and sending letters to her client base, one third of which was throwing those letters out because they were over sixty-five. That's 30% of her mailing that was going in the garbage. Of the thousands she spent on mailings, she might as well have lit a third of that money on fire.

I told her she absolutely had to split her list and advertise to that 30% separately, or just move on without them. By the next time I talked to her she had virtually eliminate Medicare to the point where it accounted for only 3% of her patients.

Collecting your Data

Of course, you need a way to gather all this data. I use a very scientific approach that I call . . . the intake form. That's part of the beauty of being in the healthcare field. Your patient will write out any information under the sun for you on this intake form, and almost never question why any of it is needed. They'll give you their emergency contact, full name, health insurance, social security, date of birth—the works.

At my practice, we even ask for e-mails and cell phone numbers so we can keep in contact with them. The fact that we ask for so much information on our intake form and the fact that most doctors have now gone to EMR (electronic medical records) means that if we have to pull this information up for marketing purposes somewhere down the road, it's a homerun. Many doctors don't even know that they already have all this information right at their disposal. I see people paying marketers tons of money because they feel like they need to have a mailing list. You already have a mailing list! You don't need to collect new addresses for an e-mail campaign; you already have that! If marketers were smarter, they'd be coming to doctors for our lists. They'd find out it's against the law for us to sell our lists off to anyone else, but we can definitely use them for ourselves.

We not only have our own giant lists, but we can narrow them down. We can target them by age group, by likes and dislikes—essentially any relevant category. It's a surprising number of doctors who never even think to capitalize on this for marketing purposes.

Using Your Data, Finding Your Tribe

The first thing I want you to do is go to your files (or have your assistant do it if you're in a position to delegate), and chart your client demographics: their gender, age group, whether they have insurance, what time of day they come to your practice, and on which day of the week, etc. In short, narrow it down. Get as specific as you possibly can. There are a lot of other variables to throw in as well that will vary depending on your practice—find them and include them. Don't stop when you think you have enough. Tabulate what symptoms they come in with, what procedures they usually end up getting, and who refers them. And not just who is doing the referring, but whether they are in-house, through your referral network, or not.

Get those stats because if you do, you can put a marketing strategy together that will blow the roof off your practice. The simple secret is that it's much easier to target those people you find specifically than it is to target the whole world. And let me tell you, it *is* tempting to want to target the whole world—whether you're working on niche-finding or you're working on marketing. I'm certainly guilty of it, too. I often have the thought, "Everyone could use this service I'm providing."

That's perfectly human, of course. Just about every dentist I talk to says, "Everyone needs their teeth cleaned or fixed. Everyone will need a root canal at one time or another." That's true, but you know when the last time I went to the dentist was? It was about six months ago, for a teeth cleaning. Without somebody reminding you—in a way that targets you—it's not something that comes to mind every day.

So you have to stand for something. As I like to say, "If you don't stand for something, you fall for anything." If you have a well-defined niche, this will be easier. But now you have to look at who is attracted to that niche and use your powers of observation to zero in on it still further.

Now, I always hear it, so I know a lot of you are saying, "Joe, I provide a lot of different services across the board." That's fine. Once you get patients through the front door, you can, and should, sell them on your other services, but what I want you to focus on right now is the element of getting them through the front door. For that, we have to narrow down that audience as much as we possibly can. You need a theme.

Developing your Theme

Let's step off to the side for a minute and take a quick look at the clothing industry. One store you've probably seen across the country is American Apparel. Maybe you've bought clothes there too; a lot of people have. They have a theme, don't they? They stand apart; they're different. They don't have logos on their clothes, and that appeals to a certain frame of mind and a certain demographic. Those people become customers, as they wouldn't necessarily if American Apparel just said, "We're a clothing store. We sell all kinds of clothes."

As another example, let's take a look at Disney. I love Disney as an example of a really intelligently run business. Their theme is "The Happiest Place on Earth." And it's not something you can argue. You go in and you're convinced it's the happiest place on earth.

Jeep is a company that has a similar effect. They have great marketing, and I know it because it works on me as well as anybody. I drive a Jeep myself and I love Jeeps. Their theme is rugged reliability, and I fit somewhere in the demographic of people that appeals to. Do I need a new car? Sure. But I think my Jeep is awesome. To me, it's the biggest man toy you could ever have, and I love it. In short, I'm a fan of Jeep. And just like I'm a fan of Jeep, I want your patients to be fans of you. We do that by getting them to talk about your practice the same way I talk to people about my Jeep. You do that by getting your tribe to identify with your theme.

Whatever kind of doctor you are, I want you to step into the shoes of a doctor of anthropology for a minute. Remember that your tribe has its own unique culture, customs, and language. I want your practice to be themed so strongly that it becomes a part of their culture. I want your tribe of patients to come to you and say, "I need this service or procedure to be performed only by you. I only want to see you, because you're the doctor I want to take care of this exact condition."

There are many examples of great ways to do this out there, but let me tell you about one client I got on the internet just the other day. They're called the Facial Paralysis Institute. Now think about that. Facial paralysis is pretty unique. It must be ear, nose, and throat doctors who work there, and I'm sure all those ENTs are educated to work on more than just facial paralysis. But so many people are hiding out there with a relevant problem, and nobody else was really attacking that corner of the market. Within sixty days of targeting patients with facial paralysis through the various channels of internet marketing and direct mail pieces to local ENT physicians, my coaching client saw so many new people coming through the door he couldn't believe it. I'm really excited for the guy; he's hitting a homerun with this theme, and getting the patients that come in for the Facial Paralysis Institute to sign up for all kinds of other services and procedures.

In essence, I want you to give people something to talk about. Have a theme that's catchy like a song on the radio, and people will talk about you like a song on the radio. That's a very real goal that you can make happen. There is someone for everyone, and if you can target those people, they will come to you. As long as you target the correct patient for the correct service at the correct practice, you have the key to success.

Sending the Right Message

Knowing the right ways to get the message out is hugely important, but it works best in conjunction with the right message. Knowing the right message is another challenge we face in our field. As with other challenges I've mentioned, there's no one pre-set formula for success, and because this is real life so much depends on the individual person. There are definitely some hints and guidelines we can look at. Let me give you an example.

Case Study: Dr. Norton Leigh

Dr. Leigh was a dentist. Nothing extraordinary about him (I'm saying this about my business partner in the nicest way possible); he was just your standard dentist. But he was also very frugal—about as cheap as they come. He was just generally opposed to spending money on his practice, including cleaning up the way it looked, because he was confident that the only selling point he needed was that he was good at what he did.

He wasn't completely wrong about that. His patients loved him because he was an excellent dentist, and that caused cognitive dissonance for his clients. He'd lose patients, and people would talk about how his staff was below par, his office wasn't clean, and how there was never any parking for it. But still there would be people who looked past the problems because his treatment was simply so good. Sure he was still in business, but Dr. Leigh was making it incredibly difficult just for his loyal clients to stay.

When Dr. Leigh hired me and I came in, the first thing we did was a reactivation campaign, just focusing on the previous six months. At the same time, I talked to the staff, and I had a survey sent out with the reactivation campaign asking why patients hadn't come back in the last six months.

The campaign did well. Not spectacularly, but well. So I sat Dr. Leigh down, and I said, "Look at this. We're making money, but let me show you the answers we got on the survey and what I've heard from your staff." I showed him what people were unhappy with. Just to drive the point home, we did a similar campaign with patients from three years back, and got similar results.

So I devised a plan of action. We would team up with the parking lot, and offer a parking voucher for anyone that comes to the office. Once we pushed it through, looked at the numbers, and made a deal with the parking lot, it turned out to be a homerun. Why hadn't he done this years earlier? Dr. Leigh's numbers flew off the charts because of that one simple change. We used his demographic information to design a campaign and locate a problem, and we found a clear way to market that addressed said problem.

Now, don't get me wrong. His office still wasn't clean, and his staff was only a little better. But for parking, people went crazy, and I successfully defended myself in the $70,000 challenge in the space of only three days. For him, my fee was definitely justified because he ended up making it back times ten. It's always a good feeling to know the real reason people aren't coming in.

For me, the biggest lesson to take away is that you don't always know what's wrong with your practice, and sometimes the best way is to ask your patients. All we asked Dr. Leigh's patients to do was fill out a survey for us, and the information we got back was a real treasure. That caused him to do some important things right. Dr. Leigh happened to be a good dentist. I've known people who were absolutely horrible practitioners, yet their clinics were absolutely packed with patients. It all depends on whether or not you know how to bring people through the door.

In the dental world especially, I often have clients complain to me about a competitor who is more successful but shouldn't be, because he doesn't have the same training and skills. In the end I tell them, "Well, he has a waiting room packed with patients; he's paying his staff well, and he's meeting his debts to private investors." That's the real bottom line.

I'd like you to learn that lesson from Dr. Leigh's experience, and I also want you to take to heart how much that survey helped us to solve the problem. Surveys explain an awful lot about what you're doing— and about what you think you're doing but really aren't. These days, I recommend that practitioners have patients start with a first-impressions survey after their initial visit. If you can't get people to do it, it may be worth it to use an incentive of some amount off the copay to ensure participation. In the end, it's usually well worth the fifty bucks or so that you take off. You need to find the problems that are holding you back.

For you, maybe a deal on a copay or on some extra services people need will be the magic element. It's different for every practitioner. In a lot of cases, you won't know what it is until you ask.

Medicare

I'll admit it, I have a personal grudge against Medicare as a revenue source. People on Medicare need medical attention as much as anyone, but the simple fact is that if you want to grow your practice as a business, going with a lot of Medicare is just not the most profitable choice.

That's for most people. If you're in a part of the country where Medicare is paying eighty dollars, but the other companies are only paying fifty, or where people who come to see you can only afford twenty, you know it. There are places where it makes sense. But in the bigger cities, that is not going to be the case. If I work with someone in an area where Medicare is the biggest provider, I concentrate on bringing in more Medicare patients. It also depends on your demographic. If you're in the middle of Palm Beach, Florida, and you're surrounded by retirees, then obviously that's all you're going to get.

All the same, we can't entirely ignore that Medicare exists. We sometimes have to grapple with the documentation issues it causes, and the loss of productivity caused by the mandated thorough documentation required in order to receive reimbursement. In my experience, most practitioners and therapists do not make a point of documenting everything properly. This is something you truly need to have a system for. If a staff member of a physical therapy clinic did all of the required paperwork, they could save their practice owner $12,000 a month.

I see a lot of practitioners who only do haphazard documentation, maybe because they're a one-man show or just don't want to put in the effort. When the insurance companies see the results of that, the clinics don't get paid. So I never lose a chance to express to my staff and partners that we have to document thoroughly and that this is how we get paid. The more you write, the better it is. The more you explain and justify what you're doing per treatment, the less chance you have of losing that paycheck.

And I've seen things change over the twelve years I've been in practice. When I started, a lot of notes could be summarized as, in essence, "John came in with a sprained ankle. John had a good day." You'd maybe add in a flow sheet of what exercises he did, and that was enough. That's not true at all anymore now that requirements are so detailed.

I talk to a lot of people who are fantastically talented specialists, but they end up making significantly less than they could because when they make submissions to Medicare or for Medical Necessity to an insurance company, the results are not good. They get responses back enumerating every instance where they didn't document doing everything they've billed for. It ends up delaying payments and even requiring refunds.

Sometimes you don't even get a payment, and all your work is lost.

I can tell you that we physical therapists are often terrible with notes. Well, as a practical matter, if you don't want to deal with documentation at all, the only way to do it is to be a physical therapist's assistant instead of a physical therapist. This is true for the other healthcare disciplines I advise as well. I admit, it's a problem for me too, but as soon as I realize I'm getting directly paid for my notes, they suddenly become very detailed.

Alternatives to Medicare

How do we, as professionals with our goals set on a cash-based practice, work towards finding a way to swerve around the Medicare trap? Can we work within the framework and remain cash-based?

Consider the population of people barely too young to collect Medicare. It could be a fantastically lucrative niche for someone to settle into if they targeted people from 50 to 65. Not only are they not collecting Medicare, but they are old enough to be more prone to medical conditions, and have been working a job long enough that they will have more disposable income or better paying insurances.

The number of baby-boomers in the marketplace now who are willing to spend money on their health and well-being is great, but I see the challenge for the entrepreneurial-minded practitioners in targeting those niches in that group who will be good customers, rather than relying on Medicare to dictate your fee for services.

One of my recent clients has a side business in which she deals with a geriatric population—generally in their late seventies or early eighties. She wanted a cash-based practice, so I put a simple question to her. "What are older people interested in?"

She happened to mention fitness. What came to my mind immediately was the Silver Sneakers Fitness Program. If you haven't heard of it, it's pretty much what it sounds like, a program of fitness workshops for seniors. So I suggested she adapt that idea for her own specialty of physical therapy. Why not do an affordable group therapy program for seniors who already love her as her loyal customers? We had that central idea, and we wanted to go with it. However, we kept going back to the problem of price point. She was worried about it, and it ended up taking us three months to implement the strategy because we needed to set that point correctly.

Eventually we found one that worked for people, and kept the workshops affordable. I won't say what we settled on because I don't want to give away my client's specific business practice, but for argument imagine a number. Then say people come in four times a week for a twenty-person class. It's easy to imagine she could start making some respectable money. I feel like my client deserves a lot of credit for this one, and she's pulling in around $1600 extra on the side each month now as a reward. That's money that you can take and invest back into your business to help it grow so you can finally drop that day job.

As a healthcare provider, you are (or should be) a trusted figure, and trust is a hugely important factor for the baby boomer population. As with everything, you'll have to use your creativity, but there are fantastic ways out there to use what is normally seen as the Medicare population to build a successful practice.

Chapter Five

The Art of Billing

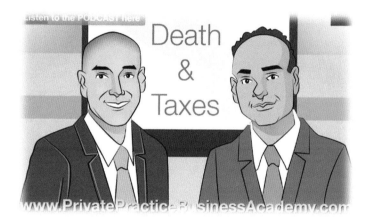

"If you cannot do great things, do small things in a

great way."

– Napoleon Hill

There are many billing services out there, and when you start out, you should probably take advantage of this fact rather than trying to handle this task yourself. I tell people to outsource it when they're just starting out, because the focus now really has to be on growing the practice. If you're concerned about who you're outsourcing to—including a billing company—you shouldn't hesitate to interview them just as you would an employee. Call them and ask questions. The people you are talking to will have an impact on your financial future. Look into your needs and the services provided. Maybe a national company doesn't fit your needs, and you need something that is local.

Once you have enough patients and your practice has grown enough to accommodate and justify the process, bring billing in-house. Eventually, it will cost you less to set up an in-house billing process than it does to pay someone else, and knowing when that moment is comes down to good, old-fashioned cost/benefit analysis. Some billing companies actually have services where they travel to your practice and train in-house staff.

Whichever way you're doing it, the most important question is whether you know your billing. You shouldn't give billing away so much that you can't keep an eye on it, and I could tell you horror stories of people who did. It's a part of the big idea that you should always be deeply familiar with every aspect of your practice, but only spend your own time doing what needs to be done by you.

Getting the wrong billing company can be one of the worst mistakes you make. If they don't know what they're doing, don't do the correct follow-up, or sign contracts with you that tie you up for years with the wrong insurance company, it could be a nightmare. It's a tough decision to make, because if you don't do your research, a bad billing company could cripple your practice before it starts.

A fair billing company will usually charge you 5-8%. And as long as the company does things aboveboard and the fees are less than what it would cost you to move billing in-house, a billing company makes perfect sense. But when the shift happens and it becomes more cost efficient to move billing in-house, a lot of practitioners are still afraid to do it. It could have to do with a cultural taboo of dealing directly with money, but many practitioners are simply unwilling to learn billing.

If you leave it to the philosophy that, "Oh, my office manager knows about that; she'll have to take care of it," that can lead to a nightmare. It actually happened to a client of mine about two years back. He's a chiropractor who decided to join a health and wellness group. He was doing really well. At the time, he was in-network with a lot of different insurances, and, without his knowing, his office manager took him off every single one of the insurances and made him out-of-network. But when the check came in, she paid him the in-network fee. Most of the time, he wasn't even getting paid due to the deductible, so he was seeing people for free.

She would pay him a fraction of what the patients paid for their treatment, and simply pocket the rest. It was insane, and she managed to get away with this for three years. He was too scared to go against her because of how long she'd be with him, and unwilling to investigate the problem because, well, you know how tough insurances are these days. But the real problem was that he was too scared to admit the fact that he just didn't want to learn this.

Obviously, she was prosecuted. She went on the run for a bit, got caught, and went for jail. It turns out that the criminal worked under aliases and pulled her scam in different states. She would go to jail, get out in two years, and do the whole thing again.

She was obviously a despicable individual, but I still blamed my client completely. He should have known better and been on top of his own business. I made him promise that if I worked with him, I never wanted to hear a single complaint about money. These days he's doing exceptionally well, because that crook he hired did him a favor and taught him that out-of-network pays more than in-network. It was a very expensive lesson, but he learned it.

Billing is an area where the general rule still applies that if you know a lot about a subject, the better your relationship will be with the person you hired to do it.

Starting Your Own Cash-Based Practice

The cash-based model is, of course, what this book is primarily about. My assumption is that you want as much of a cash-based practice and supplementary revenue streams as possible, though the advice I give is good for anyone with a clinic. The idea of a cash-based model is a hot topic lately, but it's not necessarily a thoroughly understood one. Just the other day, I overheard a pediatrician at a wedding go on at length about starting a cash-based practice . . . but he had no idea how. The key is knowing your value. If you know that and capitalize on it, you can leave insurance as far behind as you like, because people will be willing to pay for you.

Everyone assumes that they are the best. And that's good; it's a healthy way to think. But it's not enough. The mindset has to be not just "I'm the best," but "How do I get people to pay me for being the best?" A lot of healthcare practitioners I've talked to don't know where to start because they simply don't know what their value is.

Your average-joe practitioner without a plan knows that he or she is good, but couldn't answer that big question of "What's my value?" So they copy other people. They cut and paste. If they see some other guy charging a hundred dollars, they decide they're going to charge a hundred dollars too. They don't try to make any classification, or discern any difference. At that point, if you pointedly ask that practitioner "Why are you worth a hundred bucks?" the answer you're going to get is something along the lines of, "Well, that's what the other guy charges."

I want you to ask yourself two questions. Why should somebody give you that hundred bucks? And why should you only charge a hundred? If you're as good as you'll probably say you are, you probably should be charging more than a hundred dollars. If your sessions are very short, though, it might not be feasible to charge that much. In general, you want to fight the temptation to undervalue yourself. You can't just follow other people; you need a system for knowing how much you are worth and why.

When Lisa Holland branched out into starting a practice as her own business, she moved out of general physical therapy into Yoga therapy specifically. Yoga was something she had a passion for, something she could position herself as an expert in, and something she could also corner her local market in. And largely because she was targeting one segment of the population rather than everybody and their mother, her business boomed. Needless to say, that's something that you want to be able to do as well. And that's where the vital element of finding your niche comes in.

Fees

Of course, when we say you have a cash-based practice, it carries the implication that people will be able to pay with credit cards as well. The ability to take credit card payments comes with fees, but it's necessary to be able to provide that service. The fees are going to differ slightly by company, so you may want to shop around a bit. If you're just starting out, you probably want to use a reader that can attach to a cell phone or tablet PC; these are quite inexpensive and connect with one of several online services such as Square to allow you to take payments.

If you run a client's credit card, you want to make sure you have that card saved. It really makes it easier to charge copays to customers who return for future treatment. (Legally, you must have the patient's consent in a written contract to automatically charge their credit card). I hate to see people from practices chasing after people for copays. It even happens that things get busy, and people end up walking out the door without ever paying. With the credit card on file, this is no longer a loss. I've seen practices turn around just based on the losses stopped by keeping credit cards on file.

Not long ago, I spoke with Tom Cooley, a thirteen-year veteran of the credit card processing field, and president of Priority MD, an application that handles secure and compliant billing for medical practices. Tom explained to me that one big change in the card processing industry that everyone will have to take note of is the conversion to something called EMV (Euro Mastercard Visa) or the "chip and pin" card.

This is a more secure system than the one in the magnetic stripe cards that we were using and everyone who takes credit card payments needs to be equipped to process them.

This means change for us, but it doesn't necessarily mean bad news. As Tom explained, "At the core of this changeover is a shift in liability for the chargeback." What does that mean for you? Well, as things were, if a patient paid for something at your practice with a credit card, forgot about it, and tried to reverse the charge with his credit card, you as the merchant were responsible for the money. The new system is so secure that if a chargeback is approved, the issuer will be responsible for refunding the money. You're now off the hook.

The pain of change is very real, so it makes sense to know when a big, unavoidable change like this is coming down the road. That's why I like the idea of hiring out a company like Tom's if you're not already set up to handle the details of card payments on your own. As he explained, "We've set up a streamlined model that practices that implement easily and without a lot of advanced calculus in figuring out what the fee structure actually is."

Tom charges a flat fee of 2.5% and ten dollars per month, with no extra line items. The lower-than-usual transaction fee means that for most people the ten dollar bill is easily saved back, and covers their HIPA-audited product that takes care of keeping the card on file. Priority MD provides a card reader that's essentially free—it costs $99, but is refunded with the first $99 of fees.

I've been very happy with Tom's services, and I think Priority MD is a great solution for practices of any size. If you're interested, check out the interview I did with him at

http://privatepracticebusinessacademy.com/priorit ymd/

Understanding the Insurance Companies

Dealing with insurance companies tends to be a big pain point, because people don't feel like they have what they need to negotiate with them. With them, it's a constant fight. Almost everyone ends up losing more time than they want with insurance companies.

In brief, insurance companies are a huge time suck. That's why we're talking about growing a cash-based practice. But at the same time, it's important to remember that some insurance pays very well. So why wouldn't you charge them when you can? It doesn't make sense to dismiss a source of revenue completely. But in general, getting a payment from them takes weeks. It's far from the ideal situation where you would be paid immediately for a service you've performed.

Nobody wants to have to wait the six to eight weeks it can take insurance companies to pay, all the while knowing, as they sometimes never pay at all, the whole business is a giant crapshoot. And it's getting to be more and more that way, with the insurance business itself going into a spiral. With that being said, should you still take the time to understand how insurance companies work and how to deal with them? The answer is a definite yes, and not the least because insurance companies are some of the best business models out there.

Most people don't look at it that way. They like to say how much they hate them. Personally, I think of insurance companies like banks. Banks are also some of the best businesses out there, and most people don't even realize that they're businesses.

You open an account with the bank, and start making deposits there every two weeks when you get your paycheck. So what does the bank do with the money? There's no actual money in the bank. They take that money and they invest it in other branches, in real estate, etc. It's called "fractional reserve banking," and it means that the bank always has far less actual money available to it than the sum of its deposits. They can do it because they know that all their depositors are unlikely to demand all their money in cash all at once.

That's basically what the insurance company does as well. People pay into the insurance plan, and the insurance company invests it in other things. Their business isn't helped by giving back all the money you've paid in every time there's a claim, so of course they want to justify every claim to make sure it's legitimate. That's why there are so many steps to go through, and why they make you jump through so many hoops to get paid. It's a pain to deal with when we're trying to get paid by insurance companies, but that doesn't mean we can't learn from it. Try to keep that same mentality that insurance companies have when thinking about your own practice.

Dr. Joseph Simon

Banks and insurance companies have the systems mindset down pat. They're using great systems, and if you can think along those lines, you can use their philosophy to your advantage. Like banks and insurance companies, we want to make sure we have reliable, recurring revenue; we want to make sure we invest that revenue correctly in other things, and we want to make sure we cycle our patients through our businesses and other businesses so we keep generating that income.

So don't just hate them for what they do and call them crooks, like some practitioners do. Realistically, they have a system in place that we can apply to our own work. But as with Medicare, and as is generally good practice, everything should be as well-documented as possible. If you're working with insurance, you no doubt know about the new challenges of ICD-10, and how payments could take up to six months. No doubt you've already experienced this delay, and maybe a corresponding dry period. This just means that a practice needs to be even stronger with its documentation and paperwork.

Years ago, I worked at a practice where it was a running joke that everyone who came in had "lumbar ridiculopathy." I had to go with it because that's what my boss told me to do. Obviously those days are long gone. ICD-10 means absolutely everything has to be documented, down to the source and site of the pain. Of course, if you're in Canada you've been dealing with it for years.

I heard of one practice, where the owner actual docked the pay of employees every time they missed documenting something that caused the practice not to be reimbursed (which, of course, can be as simple as getting the sex of the patient wrong). Now, I'm not promoting that. I do think it's a legitimate approach, but you really need the personality to pull it off. You need to be a great manager with true leadership skills—and even then, it should be a temporary measure to shock people. You don't want staff to revolt!

Case Study: Melissa Nielli

Not long ago, I spoke with Melissa Nielli, the owner of MDN Billing and Consulting services. Melissa's an expert in examining how a practice's billing works and, in her words, "Make sure everyone can get raises because there's more revenue coming in!"

The big good news is that, as Melissa put it, "billing is billing across the board . . . you can go from PT to chiropractic to gastroenterology. Once you know your basics and your modifiers, you can pretty much take it to any different specialty and just pick up the different codes you need." You're going to need to deal with them thoroughly in your billing, and for that you need systems in place.

Melissa also stressed that with the ICD-10 in place, those who don't know its system are going to need courses and training to familiarize themselves with it. And if these courses are not the best use of somebody's time, that's what we have hiring and outsourcing for. Melissa recommended Medco Consulting, for those based in New York, as a great source for courses to get people trained up to the level they need to be to handle the demands of medical billing. Similar resources are available all around the country. Above all, she stresses, thorough documentation and knowledge of your required systems is paramount.

"I encountered a practice that didn't even do insurance verification at their front desk," she recalled. "They were losing twenty-five percent of their revenue. Half of people's insurances weren't active or had no ID numbers. Until they fixed that, of course, the billers couldn't their job! I always see revenue getting lost because something like a date of birth or the sex of the patient is incorrect. Little stupid mistakes like that can cost a practice a large amount of money yearly."

It's because billing is such an exact and detail-oriented task that I stress knowing and trusting who you have doing it to do the job well. Melissa shared, "I believe in outsourcing billing because we normally work off a percentage rate. We're not getting paid hourly. We're not just collecting a check no matter what. The practitioner doesn't have to pay payroll taxes and workers' comp. And with a billing company, there's normally more than one person. So someone gets sick or quits, there's backup that there might not be for an in-house biller. And we're more knowledgeable in that I, at least, require myself and my staff to be constantly taking courses to keep up to date. Some smaller practices can't manage that."

Melissa stresses—and I strongly agree with her—that before taking someone on for a task as important as your billing, you should interview them just as you would an employee. Not that this means you have to fire anyone if you already have people on board for this (which is why she offers training services for in-house billers as well). For more info from Melissa, give

my interview with her a listen:
http://privatepracticebusinessacademy.com/mel
issanielli/

Chapter Six

Are You Busy or Productive

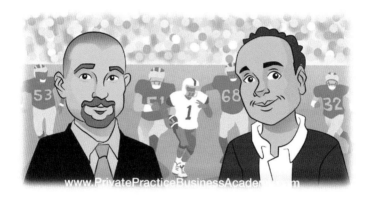

"Watch, listen, and learn. You can't know it all

yourself. Anyone who thinks they do is destined for

mediocrity."

— *Donald Trump,*
chairman of The Trump Organization,
The Trump Plaza Associates, LLC.

To be successful, sometimes you have to break outside

of the rules you're used to following. And one of those that often tends to unnecessarily bind up practices is what I call The Rule of One.

What is it? The Rule of One is the conviction a lot of people have that they can get by depending on one referral source or one marketing medium. Or even on one staff member. What I always say is The Rule of One is the most dangerous place to be.

Most private practice owners have their one referral source, and they feel like it's alright to get by with that. Maybe it's the Yellow Pages or another practice down the street. Because their practice hasn't actually closed down yet, they don't feel like they need to put the time, effort, and money into expanding their reach. It's just as dangerous to rely on only one employee to do your billing. These are things that can truly cripple a practice if they're not fixed.

Many practitioners struggle because they don't really want to fix this problem. They're not pressured to fix it, because to them, it seems to be smooth sailing. The waters may seem to be calm, but if a storm hits, that's it. What if that larger practice down the street steals all the referrals from a doctor's office because he's bought them out or started giving them kickbacks. What are you going to do when Google changes its search parameters, and you no longer have referrals coming in from the internet?

I recently consulted with a physical therapist. She has two practices, and she's been practicing for twenty-five years. She was doing amazingly because she had a doctor who referred to her on a regular basis. When she started all those years ago, she really helped him out and even paid for his office, because she knew that he would generate patients and send everybody over to her.

What that meant was for twenty-five years, this woman was coasting on the rule of one. Well, one day, all of a sudden, her friend the doctor got an offer from a hospital. They offered him a huge amount of money, and bought out his practice. And when they did it, they told him he was now only allowed to refer all of his patients to the hospital's own physical therapist.

Overnight, my client's practice went from banking tons of money, to not even boasting one patient. At that point, she called me up and said, "What do I do?" She was falling apart: she knew she had a lot of staff, a lot of overhead, and a lot of rent, and she needed to know fast how she could keep it going. Looking at the structures she had in place, it seemed to me she had about three months before she would go completely bankrupt.

But, of course, it wouldn't have been that kind of problem for her if she hadn't spent over two decades following the Rule of One. Trying to recoup that kind of cash flow that quickly is pretty tough. It's a sad story, but at that point, she had to be trying to sell a practice. And even then, few people want to buy a practice which for decades, has only had referrals from one vanished source.

It made me feel like putting a "Rule of One" stamp right on her front door as I walked out. It's a trap none of us can afford to fall into. That can be a hard lesson. And it's one that I personally learned the hard way when I started out.

At my first practice, when I was only a small, solo practitioner, I hired an administrative assistant, and she was fantastic. She learned the ropes, and she knew how to run every aspect of everything at our practice. The problem arose when she became pregnant.

Now, most people who have children understand that for the first three months of a pregnancy, the mother is usually either sleeping or pretty tired. And for those first three months our administrative assistant was out of it. We lost so much money during that time, and especially at the size of my operation, that really hurt. It crushed me, because that was all I had to live on.

And so when she came back, I had a realization. I had ninety days to figure out how to avoid the same problem happening a second time. I needed to hire somebody and train them on everything that she could do, because I knew she would be gone again – and there was no way of knowing how long her maternity leave would be. We managed to do it, but without that initial shock of her first absence we may not have learned the lesson in time to avoid potential disaster.

Even today, we try to work this lesson into every aspect of our practice. Quite simply, putting all of your stock into one person isn't very smart; you need a plan for when that person isn't there. It sounds simple, but fighting against the Rule of One is a constant battle. Quite frankly, the Rule of One is comfortable. Once you've got something going and the waters are calm, you just don't want to think about it. Even when the dangers are pointed out to them, most people will argue with you. I can't count the number of times I've been told, "I don't have money to hire a second person," or, "I don't have money to use another referral source," or, "I don't have money to market something else."

Well, in this case, P. T. Barnum was right. When a man told him he couldn't afford to advertise, Barnum's simple response was, "Sir, you can't afford NOT to advertise." It's just as true when you're running a health practice as a circus. Because I guarantee that if you don't prepare, you'll be worse off when the storm hits. Because now, you're going to have to spend more money—and that will be money you're losing rather than money you're investing.

As hard a life lesson as it can be, it happens over and over again. Practitioners just keep falling into the trap of feeling like as soon as they get the one they want, they're set. And they never stop coming to regret it later on.

The 95-5 Rule—Managing Your Time

Here's another concept that I want to make sure is understood, and it relates closely to the Rule of One, because it directly has to do with how you spend your time most efficiently. You always want to concentrate on the 5% of things that is most efficient to your time and will pay you the most return. The other 95% of things you have to delegate and assign to staff or virtual assistants.

Now, if you're not up to 95-5, it's not necessarily an immediate disaster. That's a goal we're looking towards. Maybe you're at 75-25. Even with only 25% on your plate and 75% being delegated out, you're not doing badly . . . but is there more you could outsource so you can focus even more on your own wheelhouse? The best way to start is by breaking down what others should be doing and what you should be doing. Let's take the example of cleaning the bathroom.

I'm sure you have one in your office. But cleaning it shouldn't be a part of your five percent.

The way to look at it is in terms of your hourly wage. What do you want to get paid for an hour? That's a question I ask everybody. Usually people start breaking down statistics and they come up with a figure. Maybe $105 or $220 per hour. I say, "Sure. But what would you *want* to be paid for the hour?"

Maybe you'll say you want to get paid $1000 for the hour. Alright—so let's stick to that! How likely do you think a thousand-dollar employee would be to clean your office's bathroom? People I talk to agree, and I'm sure you do too, that's best delegated to someone making ten to fifteen dollars per hour. So let's delegate cleaning the bathroom rather than doing it ourselves.

That's an obvious example (hopefully!), but you have to break down each of your tasks in the same way. Is that worth a thousand-dollar-an-hour employee's time? If not, you want to try to find a way to delegate it to somebody else.

Now, I know you're probably not making that thousand dollars every hour. Probably less than 1% of practitioners are. But that's the goal. We all want to get there. And to do that, we need to start budgeting our time as if it's worth what we feel it should be. If you need a mantra when you're budgeting your time, keep thinking that's what your time is worth, and that you need to protect your time. That's what I do. And everything that's not in my top 5%, where I'm creating, networking, and making the business grow, then I try to outsource it and give it to staff to do.

Case Study: Albert

I have a client named Albert who I think provides a great example of this concept. The man has five kids and a superhuman wife who is willing to do just about anything for him. Albert works a lot. He'll go into work at 7:00 am and get done at 7:00 PM. But then he stays at the office until midnight working on his practice. That means he's working in his practice for twelve hours a day, then working ON his practice for another five. And that's horrible time management—maybe the worst I've ever seen.

It didn't take me long to see problems here. The man was killing himself with work and spending no time with his family. Our first meeting became one about how to take that time he was staying in the office between seven and midnight, and give those five hours back to Albert's family.

We started working with the staff. We found out that between eleven and one, things tended to slow down. So we decided during that time, instead of chatting with the staff, he would leave it with them and go to Starbucks. If he was a solo practitioner, I would have said to close the office during that time, because it's slow anyway.

Look at the numbers, find when the slowest time is, and block that off for yourself. That becomes the time when you work on your practice and not in your practice. That alone makes a huge difference. These days, when the end of the day comes at seven, Albert can go home. That was just week one of me working with Albert, and that week one paid huge dividends.

The Thirty-Minute Increment

Making the kind of change that I led Albert to make is a huge challenge, and a lot of it has to do with mindset. Working the way Albert was is something people feel like they have to do, and if they're not doing it, they start to feel guilty. When they're not working hard, they feel like they're not helping the business. So they like that feeling of "busy."

But when you're running a business, feeling like you're busy doesn't always mean that you're actually being productive. And that's a huge message that is sometimes a real challenge to get through to people. So when I sit down with a client, I try to break down their entire day with them into thirty minute increments. I send them a piece of paper to fill out showing what they do with their day in thirty minute blocks, and even filling in that sheet of paper tends to present a challenge for them.

A lot of people tell me they can't do it. I say, "You know what I charge you for the month? I can break down into thirty minute blocks all that time that you're paying me for. Do you want to lose money or make money?" And then they usually do it—because what I'm giving them is not a justification for busywork but a legitimate analogy. You're supposed to be getting paid for the time you are spending on your practice, so you should know how you spend it.

When people actually break down their day, they're usually surprised to see that a lot of things they spend their day doing actually consist of busywork. They're doing unnecessary things or work that should be delegated just to keep themselves occupied. Everyone likes to do the easy stuff first, right? Well, that's true of my practitioner clients as well. They tend to want to spend their time doing extraneous, easy things that make them feel like they're busy doing something, or accomplished once they've finished it.

Sometimes on those certain days when there really isn't anything to do, instead of relaxing or just being in the present and enjoying not doing anything, these people are busy plugging away doing nothing of importance. In their mind, any moment of idleness means they're not getting anything accomplished. But what they really don't have accomplished is their goals. They don't know what they're supposed to be doing during the day. The reason is by and large that these people never sat down and figured out what 5% of things they should be doing, and what 95% should be delegated.

When Do You Take on an Employee?
The team you surround yourself with from the start doesn't necessarily have to be staff. But eventually, your practice will probably get big enough that you will want to consider hiring. You need to be empirical in terms of justifying that hiring.

Look at your numbers, and make sure that the gains of taking on an employee would be greater than the losses. Find a standard where that threshold is met. Do you need forty or fifty patients per week? Twenty? It will depend on the economics of your own practice.

Often people just know when they've hit the number of patients where they're busting at the seams and can't take on any more work personally. When you feel like that, and there's more work than you can do, sit down and crunch the numbers to see if you can support finding help.

That help might come in the form of an assistant, or of another practitioner. It might even turn out to be more useful for you to bring in a strategic partner than an employee. If you're a dentist, bringing on an orthodontist can give you both a referral source and somewhere to send extra patients coming through your door. Another example would be a physical therapist partnering with or hiring a message therapist.

In the beginning it will be tough, because you will need to fill that new person's schedule up. You're going to basically hand that person your schedule, and then it will be your job to fill your own schedule up again! Put a training period in place and go through it step by step.

Chapter Seven

Being a Leader

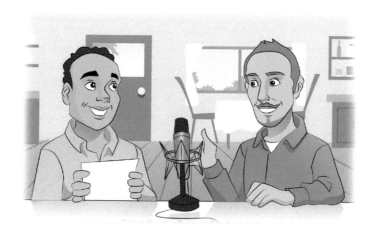

"A leader is one who knows the way, goes the way, and

shows the way."

– John C. Maxwell

Leadership is a big challenge for a lot of owners. I meet a lot who simply want to crawl back and be a worker bee again, because they find leadership intimidating.

But it shouldn't be. Being a leader doesn't mean you're superhuman, and it doesn't mean you have to be the smartest guy in the room. It doesn't even mean you're the most talented treating clinician in the office. It means you're someone other people can follow. The mere fact that you have had the courage to start and run your own practice means a lot.

Being an effective leader and understanding the keys to management in private practice are not traits you are born with. Or are you? I certainly wasn't. I had to learn the hard way—and I didn't do it overnight. Everything from reading book after book on management and training, to seeing how the practices that I coach operate on a daily basis, to real experiences in my own practice have made me the leader that I am.

But these skills are not inborn. You need to create margins, train your staff properly, keep your finances open with your staff, and have open monthly meetings if you want to keep your business running, and running well. What's more, you need to be assertive. I've seen owners avoid confrontation on a daily basis just to keep the status quo, and that can be deadly. I get a lot of kickback on that point about financial information, but I think that transparency is very important. Share your financial information with your staff.

You have to keep things scaled. I own multiple practices with my strategic partners included, and if I were to add a lot more, I would need a management team on board to help with the added logistics. It all goes back to outsourcing when you need to and managing your time alongside your people.

But on an individual level, a lot of managing people uses the same interpersonal skills that you develop as a healthcare professional. It's remarkable how far you will be taken simply by listening effectively. People forget that diamonds can really be in your own backyard. If you see a person not progressing, give them incentive to progress. Challenge them, support them, coach them. It may not work, and you may need to dismiss them. But it only makes you a better leader and manager—and helps your practice—to try.

In a lot of cases you already have the talent you need. I hear owners complaining all the time about all areas of their staff, not just professional but administrative. Personally, I'll always lean more towards training. The saying I give them is, "Let's do less complaining and more training." In training, as in everything, once you have an effective system down, you can replicate it and keep going with it as you grow.

Who you hire is very important, not just to how you manage them, but to the customer experience. And, of course, having easy people to work with will make it much easier to do your job of leadership well. The key is the person.

How do You Hire?

Most private practitioners hate hiring. They hate it so much that they try to avoid having to do it at any cost. But there are good reasons to always be hiring and to make sure you train everyone thoroughly and completely. In fact, the number one reason I see that employees go bad is that they were improperly trained. I have a ninety-day training process at my business, but

I'm not afraid to get rid of people who aren't contributing anything after even two weeks.

Having a mentor and a system in place when you hire is very important, in my view. If you just decide to roll the dice and put an ad in the paper saying you need someone you can teach how to answer the phones, then you're making the same mistake that has personally cost me literally hundreds of thousands of dollars.

There are a lot of practice owners out there right now who have poisonous employees on board, and they don't have the courage or ability to get rid of them. People like that get their jobs because their bosses weren't hiring carefully.

My short answer to the question of how to hire is that you have to *always* be hiring. I literally mean that this process should be non-stop. You should always have an interview coming up. Does this mean you should have an ad for new people running on a consistent basis? Yes. I think you should have an ad up at least every three months for a different position, from your professionals to your support staff, and even summer internships.

Why? There are two reasons. First, your current staff is going to want to know why you are interviewing. Obviously, to see if there's anybody else out there you want to hire. This will keep them on their toes. They'll know you're constantly looking for someone who is better, and you shouldn't hide this; it means you want your practice to grow and to be the best.

Secondly, and most obviously, you want to find those good employees who will help your business. The kind of ad you write in order to do that is very important. You want to weed out tire-kickers and people who are just looking for something in between other jobs.

Once you get a person in, do not hire anyone at first sight, no matter how much you like them. You need to do a minimum of two to three interviews. Start with a phone interview; give them a task to complete, and then move on to the in-house interview. These all make it challenging for the interviewee, so you know anyone who completes all this wants the job and wants to work hard for the job. And the tasks that they complete will give you a better understanding of them as a worker.

There are a million reasons why a person might not work out. Maybe they don't have the typing skills, or the phone skills, or the organizational skills you need. Maybe they can't answer your questions. That's why you need to have so many levels of interview, and that's why you always need to have another interview lined up.

If you do this, then by the time you bring someone by for the in-house interview and see them interacting with your essential staff members, you will really have a strong feeling for whether or not this person will be the right fit for your practice.

Even after all that, no matter how well you do it, you may still make a mistake. Even I do from time to time. No matter how well that candidate goes through the interview, the way they interact with customers may not be a good fit. So put a ninety-day probationary period into effect.

"Hire slow; fire fast," sums up my position on this. If they do not have a good personality or tolerate training well, you have to let them go immediately. It's a huge pain point for a lot of practices because owners just don't want to spend that much time on hiring. It's something they hate working on. I'm different because I love it, and when I come in as a partner, I'm very insistent that this is something we have to do.

Put Together a Team

When you're starting a practice, even if it is a minimal one, you are going to want to have a team in place. So you find a lawyer, you find a banker, you find an accountant. You don't need to start off paying everybody from step one. But eventually this process will be one by which you become an employer. And the more programs you start offering, the more you are going to want and need to hire.

To avoid putting all your eggs in one basket, you don't want to cover everything yourself individually, and you don't want any other individual doing it either. It should go without saying that when your business grows enough, you will need to have a good staff working under you in order to support that growth.

It's been said that everyone—be it in the world of healthcare, business, or both—is one of two types of people. There's the entrepreneur who's always thinking, always working, always trying to push things further. That's me, and if you're reading this book, it's you too.

But there are also people who thrive on going to work, doing their job, going home, and turning the work-related part of their brain off. You want a work environment where these people can thrive and contribute as well.

Basically, you're interviewing a bunch of people. See which people will work well with you, and which people will give you good, honest advice. See which one educates you the best, and that's the one you keep onboard. You might end up going through two or three accountants, or two or three bankers. It's always good to know as much as possible.

So find this team. It is the number one referral network that you are going to need. And you are going to need services as well. Now, I've recently moved on to my sixth accountant. And you too are going to change team members as well, as your practice grows. The sooner you assemble a team that is valuable to you, the better.

You want people who you can be honest with, and who will realize that you're all in it together as far as making sure the practice grows. You want people who will react to a setback by doubling down, sticking onboard, and working still harder. It's not worth it being afraid that people will jump ship, because if they're going to do it, they usually do it right away. I tell people, "Out of respect, let us know when you know if you're going to be leaving." And beyond that, it's a factor out of your control.

I have a system that I go through for hiring people, but like anything, it is not always certain. Sometimes we hire a rockstar, and sometimes we hire a dud. I am quite confident, though, that we are hiring rockstars a lot more often, and when we get a dud, we know how to dispense of them while doing minimal damage to the practice.

Successful hiring means finding a happy medium. Someone too fresh may not sufficiently know what they're doing, but someone too seasoned may not be able to adapt well. It's a constant balancing act.

In my case, I own a few practices outright, and I'm a partner in a few others as well. Because I've delved into the business end of things so deeply, I've implemented that 95-5 rule very strongly, and I don't actually treat patients anymore when my time is best spent handling the business side of things.

It's always a big challenge for me to have to work with a clinical director who has no background in business, marketing, or sales. It's become a pet peeve of mine, because it's something that could be avoided in the hiring process. Of course, I was a staff member myself in the past, and I know it can be difficult to see one side from the other. So in the last few years, I've learned to stop micromanaging, trust my team, and know when the right time is to step in and say, "Alright, guy. This is how you do this."

For a lot of practices, the staff is one of the biggest expenses, second only to the rent. If you choose wisely, they will justify that expense and be your most important asset. Some big companies will go to the expense of hiring and training employees, then offer them a lump sum of three thousand dollars to leave. Why? Because those employees who don't take the payoff are really dedicated to the company, and these are going to be the only truly valuable ones. They would lose well over three thousand on a poor employee. For more information about this model, I recommend reading about the online shoe company Zappos, and their founder, Tony Hseih. It's a story I was able to take a lot of lessons from.

Errant Employees

When you have a practice, and you train practitioners to work under you, you're running an inherent risk of seeing some of them break off to do it on their own. It's a scary thought. Not only are you losing a part of your own practice that could be hard to replace, that part is now actively working against you in his or her own practice. But the fact is, some people are entrepreneurial-minded. They should be. In my opinion, intelligent people are more likely to be, and if you run your practice well as a business, it's going to foster that atmosphere.

So it may be counterintuitive, but I personally think it's a great thing if your staff members end up branching out on their own. It means you're doing something right. And let's not forget: we're in healthcare. The more competent and skilled people we can get out there helping people with their health problems, the better. As long as they're not directly taking your clients, the more the merrier. Needless to say, one practitioner can't treat everybody. When all is said and done, people are going to move on no matter what. People who learned well are going to pay their respects to the one they learned from. Of course, if you were that mentor, that can only come back to benefit your own standing and reputation. It only brings you up higher—and it means that you've been the leader rather than the follower.

As Donald Trump Would Say: "You're Fired!"
If you have people on staff, sooner or later you are going to have people working under you whom you need to fire. Sometimes a simple philosophy like "Hire slow; fire fast" doesn't cover enough to make clear

exactly when you need to do that. This is an unpleasant subject for a lot of owners I work with because it makes them feel like they are being too mean, but you can't be a business owner with a practical policy of never dismissing an unsatisfactory employee.

I'm working with a clinician right now whose front-desk associate just should not be in that position. I've said this many times, but firing her is a tough sell, because she's a friend of the owner's. So we go back and forth on the question. It's a clear decision for me, looking from the outside in, but not for someone who knows her.

So, of course, it's not always an easy decision. The example above also illustrates just as well that hiring your friends can be a risky proposition. And, of course, we're all human. We get emotionally tied people.

For example, I consulted with a practice that was trying a new strategy for how they answer the phone and interact with people. We gave them a whole script for it. We would call and pretend to be a patient asking for these services. But we found the office manager, who had been with the practice for twenty-five years, was so hard-set in her ways that she didn't want to change. She didn't care what some kid came in and told her, that kid being me.

My gut feeling was that she would be dead-set against it. When I had come in to do the training, I could see from her face and her mannerisms that she just didn't care in the least. I even confronted her about it, and she blew me off. As you can imagine, I told the owner, but he was reluctant to do anything because she had been there for so long.

Well, as it happens, we record our calls when we test-dial a practice to try out their phone-answering system. It's a very easy call; we're basically asking to give them money. She picked up on two of three calls, and every other word out of her mouth was "No." She seemed to be making it as difficult as possible for the patient to do business with them.

When we played those tapes back to the practice owner, he was mortified. There she was essentially refusing money for the practice, and she didn't care because she was still going to get the same paycheck with the same vacation time as always. Her hours and income would remain the same even if the owner struggled; she was too comfortable.

In the end, she was let go. It was a hard step for the owner to take, but she was costing him money. He struggled for maybe a week or two as he tried to figure things out, but then he started to work out other ways of making things happen. Without her there, he realized how slow she was at doing some stuff—including some things that could simply be outsourced or phased out. In ways that he didn't realize when he fired her, that dismissal ended up saving him a ton of money. He basically gave himself a raise. Her salary was taken, chopped up, and brought to different services.

But everyone is guilty of being too reluctant to fire sometimes when the human element comes in. I certainly have been in the past. That office manager of mine I told you about earlier was the same way; I thought she was the be all and end all, but it came back to bite me.

As I mentioned before, she'd been with me from the very beginning of my practice. And the big thing that she always liked to repeat was how she had worked at bigger, corporate companies in the past. She would always tell me, "You know, in corporate America, they do it this way . . ."

I didn't know any better at the time. I figured whatever she said must be the best way to do things. She always seemed to be busy, she was there forty-plus hours a week, and to me it really seemed like she was always trying to help me out. It wasn't as if things weren't getting done.

But one day, this office manager became really furious about something to do with her taxes. She insisted that I couldn't give her a 1099, and that everything had to be on her salary. Which wasn't what the accountant had recommended. She pulled that "corporate America" line on me again, but this time I had done the research. And the non-salary expenses we were talking about did have to be put on her salary—*if* she was part of a company of *over* fifty people.

We only had about ten people working in our business. So I told her, "Until your name's on the front door, we are going to do it my way." She was irate at that comment, but I was dead right. I had actually done the research. And at that point, I started to realize that she just tended to make a lot of stuff up in order to get her way.

Then it became a matter of principle. I started to do my research on everything she told me. A lot of what she said was incorrect. When I approached her about it, she became very defensive, and then she started to poison the other employees against me.

Eventually, she showed up one day really dressed up. She said, "Oh, I'm going to go visit this

106

other doctor today because he asked that I stop by to drop off some information about the clinic." I let it go, but it was obvious to everyone that she was blatantly lying, and was in fact going for an interview.

She got this other job, and gave us two weeks' notice. Other employees were worried because they thought of her as knowing how to do everything. But at that point, she basically stopped working. She came in when she wanted to, then left earlier than her shift. Why was I keeping this person here for two weeks who wasn't helping us and didn't want to be here?

So at that point I told her, "I think we're pretty good. Why don't you take the time off and have a little vacation before you start your new job?" She was shocked. We assumed we needed all sorts of help from her. I told her this after work when there were no other employees around.

The next day, everyone was stunned that I had given her this vacation. Now the things she had said about me didn't make any sense. And when I sat down with the other assistant to go over the things that she did, we found that it wasn't very much at all! It was almost like the *Seinfeld* episode where Costanza goes around shuffling papers instead of working. That was her.

I still can't believe when I think of all the time, money, connections, and friendships that I lost because of her. It would have been crippling to my business if I didn't have the strength to start examining her claims critically, and eventually to move on. It probably took me a year to bounce back fully from every aspect of that experience—she had set up that many different things incorrectly.

Eventually, I had to let some of the people who had been friends with her go too, because she had affected their attitudes so badly. When you bring in new people you can leave the old people there if they're still poisoning the new people! It took me about two years to overhaul the staff all around. Know who is friends with whom and who hangs out with whom. Otherwise that person you've already dismissed can still remain a very expensive mistake.

If you know someone was allies with an employee whom you've had to fire, sit down with them and have a blunt conversation. They have a choice to either stay or go. But at the end of the day you have to put food on the table to feed your family. You're the one that took the risk to start a business, and they didn't. If they can't be on board with that, you have to let them go.

It can be a harsh, ruthless way of looking at it. And I feel bad when I have to dismiss someone too. But when all is said and done, they're your employees, not your friends, and not your family. You have to take care of your own friends and family.

Finding that problem employee before they can become a problem is tough. Sometimes it's even the CEO or owner. Maybe it's the middle management. But if you have a good turnover rate, employees generally won't have time to lose that spark, and you won't have time to become too dependent on one person. It's another reason to be always hiring.

If people are doing well for you, shower them with gifts. You want to do what you can to make sure they stay on board. The people who stay are the ones you can't be cheap with because they're going to see all the transition, and they're going to wonder, "Am I next?"

Chapter Eight

Sourcing Clients

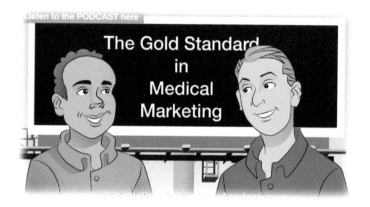

"I'm not afraid of dying, I'm afraid of not trying."

– Jay Z

If you build it, they will **not** come—unless you show them the way.

To be successful in your practice, you need to bring in new clients, and you need to make patients repeated, long-term clients. Both tasks have their challenges, but you have a broad and all-important tool your disposal: marketing.

For years, most medical practices survived with very little marketing, if any at all. They relied principally on word of mouth, or through insurance companies and HMOs that had them listed. Maybe you were even one of them. But to grow a cash-based practice in today's environment, that's simply inadequate.

Now, don't get me wrong, I think word of mouth is great. It's fantastic if you're starting a practice, and it can be a very effective way of keeping your overhead down. But sooner or later, a plateau effect is going to occur.

That plateau will appear when marketing and advertising strategies are needed, and they're just not there. You'll inevitably need to bring them in. If you've set things up correctly, word of mouth can keep going, and that's a good thing. But sooner or later marketing will have to be brought in if your practice is to grow, even if it is but one of several poles in the water.

One thing that a lot of practitioners don't appreciate, in my experience, is the difference between marketing and sales. If you've been practicing for some time and you've been relying on referrals for clients, there is a decent chance that you already had or had considered hiring a marketing person who would go around to doctors' offices to generate referrals. Chances are, this was not somebody with a degree in marketing. It was someone who understood sales.

And for you, as a cash-based practitioner, this catch-22 can rear its head again. I get people from bigger practices asking me all the time whether they should hire a marketing person. The concept is sound—it goes right along with the concept of outsourcing everything that could be better done by somebody else. But sales are going to be important to you, too, and you'll want to know if that marketing person is good at sales. Because if you are courting doctors for referrals, you've wasted a lot if that person couldn't clinch the sale and get the referral.

Most physical therapists I know shy away from the word *sales*. Many physicians like to say, "We're not salesmen. We're clinicians." That's true up to a point. But when a patient first comes into your office for a consultation, you are selling them on your service. If it's a new program you're implementing, you are selling that patient on how they are going to get better and on how long it is going to take. There's no denying it, and if you're not thinking of it that way, you're doing yourself a disservice.

You'll see that sales and marketing dovetail into each other a lot, but it's not good to confuse one for the other. As simply as possible you need marketing to drive up sales. Marketing happens when you spend time, effort, or money to help your practice. A sale happens when someone hands you money. And the first key to that is getting patients through your door.

As you'll see in the sections ahead, there are innumerable ways to market your practice—and I'm sure that you'll be able to think of some that I don't even mention in this book. But the common thread is that to be effective, your marketing must be arresting—it must make an immediate impression. If it's funny, so much the better. But whatever it is that you do, if it is memorable, it will be far more effective than the old standards of having somebody stop by with candy and a cookie-cutter sales pitch.

113

We'll start by looking at some ways to attract new clients, then look at some ways to keep the ones you have. But all of the principles I'll discuss will be applicable in a myriad of situations.

New Clients

It's common sense—or if it isn't, it should be—that patients are everything to your practice. But most practitioners neglect that sorely. They think they're some character from "Braveheart," and they practice blind archery—shooting some arrow off into the distance and hoping it hits someone. Obviously, I want you to take a different approach.

When you're starting off, landing that first client is a vital hurdle. When looking to generate new clients, you have to get into the patient's shoes and play to your strengths. That means you have to know what sort of client you're likely to get (which also plays into leveraging your data well).

A lot of practices already have clients who are very loyal (something you want for yourself), so luring them away may not necessarily be a rewarding task. Hospitals have bought up a lot of private practices and have started referring there, so you don't want to rely too much on those referrals. They've developed a sort of monopolistic business model in the healthcare field. It's a fact of life in today's medical world, and one that I constantly hear people complain about online on LinkedIn, or even in person. As a cash-based practice, you have to work against that monopoly to bring clients to your independent business.

The majority of what you do to bring in new clients is going to come down to marketing and advertising directly. Personally, I don't really even see patients in my practice who were referred by physicians. I get maybe one a month contacting me, and three a year who actually come into my office. Honestly, the majority of referrals from practices are not great ones, because that's not my client base.

I get clients by marketing to my current patients and to people I think could be good potential patients, and that's where you will be the most successful, too. The client you want to pick up is one looking for information and trying to make an informed choice. Your marketing needs to provide that information and be that choice.

We've already talked about several ways to market aspects of your business in various contexts, and we're going to talk about still more. None of them are wrong, but some may be more or less right for your individual circumstances. As I tell people all the time, I can't give you a method that is guaranteed to get you thirty clients. But I can give you thirty methods that are guaranteed to get you one client. What we as practitioners need to do is try all those ways.

I wish there was a magic pill you could take like in "The Matrix" that would generate all those clients instantaneously. But there isn't, and anyone who tells you there is, is lying. It takes a lot of work. It involves reaching out to the community, and it will probably take people seeing your name a few times before they actually make the decision to pick up the telephone or drop by for an appointment. If you take my advice and try as many reliable methods as you can, your effort will be rewarded.

115

Your Boss's Clients

I very strongly recommend not poaching that client from an employer or former employer. Simply put, that's just not cool. Your boss figured out a way to get those clients in through the front door. If there is a client who is unhappy with the services they are getting at the time, your practice is something you can mention. Obviously, as a medical professional, you become very close to people. It's a trust factor. If people trust you, you might be able to say, "Listen, I do this on the side privately. This is what it will cost." You'll land your first client immediately. It's one way to get your first person and take a test run to make sure you know what you're doing.

But the ethics of the situation really depend on the particular relationship you have with your employer. If you have a good relationship, and your employer knows about and supports your endeavor, they may be happy to send some clients your way. If you specialize in different areas, you can send referrals each other's way, and that's just good karma.

We should never be arrogant enough to forget that we don't always have the answer. It's OK to refer out. In a lot of these situations, you help the patient; you help a colleague, and you help yourself by generating goodwill and referrals for yourself down the road. Almost every practitioner I've talked to has resisted this. They feel like when they lose a patient, they are losing money. That's not always true. A networking coup can be much more valuable than one client, and every time you help a patient, you are also helping yourself.

One of my favorite quotations is from the motivational speaker and author Zig Ziegler. He said, "You will get all you want in life, if you help enough other people get what they want." I really believe that, and it's a big part of why I'm sharing my experiences with you in this book. I think the subject of our mutual relations and networking with our colleagues is one where Zig's philosophy truly applies.

Remember, you're not starting off with a claim that you're going to heal everyone of everything. As you know, that would be a big mistake. You're going to be specializing in something and shooting for a niche. If that niche isn't just the same as your employer's, you'll be able to help each other and refer clients mutually depending on whose services they need.

Networking

Never let it be forgotten that there is really nothing more to referrals than getting good information out there. Unfortunately, a lot of people I meet still live under the illusion that if they just put a sign up or are in-network with an insurance company, people will magically appear.

As you know, that's not true. We've seen how you can build awareness on the internet, and you can and should encourage it to spread by word of mouth. Probably the very best way to generate referrals is by networking.

Once people meet you, you create that like and trust factor. If you can bring that about, you'll absolutely generate more referrals than you know what to do with. You can network just about anywhere—

whether you're doing it at meetup.com or at an actual meet-up.

You can even go right to the Chamber of Commerce to see what is going on in your community. If there's an event going on, participate in that event. Will you get paid for that? No. But you have to get out there and network as much as possible. In these conversations, you're basically offering your time and services for no pay, but the networking factor alone is worth it.

There are other gurus out there who will tell you that the Chamber of Commerce is a waste of time. My response is this: you get out what you put in. The key is not thinking that each interaction you have will be an immediate client, but that each interaction will lead to another interaction. If you're going to go out and network, it only makes sense if you're going to do it right. Doing it right means actually working hard to build that like and trust. That means getting involved in your community. You can tie this into what interests you, so you're doing your own thing while at the same time building good will, getting to know people, and getting the word out about who you are and what you do. You're not getting paid for this now, but it can cause you to be paid very nicely later on.

Look at what other successful people are doing to build relationships in your community. Think about how these strategies apply to you. Not everyone's religious, but if you are, make sure to build relationships at your place of worship. If you're a sports person, get involved in your favorite sport locally. If you're new to the area, don't be afraid to ask the staff at your local chamber where you can start getting involved in the community.

Do not just go and hand out business cards. Let me impress on you now: I've been to a lot of marketing seminars discussing how a business card should be laid out, and all sorts of aspects of how to get ahead on the business card front. All this is nice if you want a pretty business card, but it isn't going to get you very far ahead. Trust me, if a person wants your business card, they will ask you for your business card. And the only thing that will lead them to that point is talking to you.

Getting Involved with a Sports Niche:

Here is a step-by-step tactic I have used for the sports niche. I hope it gets your head buzzing with ideas. Getting involved with local high school, college, and even professional teams can really give a boost to your practice. If you work with athletes, this is a referral goldmine—not only in terms of the athletes themselves, but for their family members, teammates, and others in your patient's sphere. It doesn't matter what your specialty is. Even a dentist could work with college athletes.

On many campuses, a medical practitioner needs to be on the field before a game can proceed. Being that doctor can immediately boost your expertise and your standing in your community. You become the trusted doctor and healthcare mentor for those athletes, some proportion of whom are going to suffer injuries.

I've worked high school football games as an EMT, and I found that when I was there with the physician, I had two hours of time just hanging out with him or her. That's two hours of just hanging out. It's not difficult to become qualified to be an EMT, and I built great relationships with these physicians. Without fail, people refer to you because they trust you and they like you. If you act cool around them and convince them you're a fun person, it will work in your favor.

I became determined that at every football game I work, I would meet the physician, introduce myself, and try to take the opportunity to hang out. It was some of the best marketing I had ever done in my life. I didn't have to go to any offices or bang on any doors; I had two hours of this guy's undivided attention. We'd talk about everything from football (which I'm a fan of; why else would I want to work the games?) to clinical skills. It was a great angle for me. By getting the physician on the field to say, "Joe's a good guy. Let's take care of him," I generated a lot of business for myself.

If you do that as a physician rather than an EMT, of course, this is something you can get paid for, as an extra bonus. The connections you make can lead not just to referrals but to all sorts of other opportunities in sports medicine. You don't work these games in order to get a direct funnel of patients. There's nothing but your own hard work that guarantees that. You want to work with the other specialists and make yourself a piece of the puzzle. By doing that, you're making yourself an expert. And there's nothing more valuable to be than an expert.

As word spreads, people will associate you with being knowledgeable about and involved in women's tennis, high school swimming, or whatever it may be. If you work with a sports organization that uses a logo, the ability to put up a recognizable emblem is very powerful as well. If you can get a testimonial from a recognized athlete or one from a recognizable program, that's pure gold.

Mutual referrals:

Having a traditional relationship in place with a doctor is not the only way to generate clients by way of a referral. The fact that you, if you are doing things right, have niched yourself down so much will naturally mean that you encounter a lot of problems outside of your specialization. You can enter into mutually beneficial arrangements with other practitioners to refer patients who better fit each other's niches.

Not to sound too cynical, but the concept of helping people out other than their own patients is actually fairly foreign to a lot of physicians and physical therapists I know. The scarcity mindset is still ingrained heavily in many practitioners today.

If you can't treat a patient because you have no openings for appointments or because their problem is outside of your area, it's nice to remember that, in the medical world as anywhere, what goes around comes around. If you help your colleagues, they will by and large come to your help when needed as well.

Online Networking:

More than anything, networking itself is about knowing how to talk to people, and building a relationship. That's just as possible online as it is in person, and the internet has opened up an incredible number of doors to networking with people around the globe. Sites like LinkedIn and Facebook are, of course, good for more than just promoting your site and getting information out online. There's a reason they're called social networks.

The next generation of people coming up and starting in the healthcare field has an advantage that I originally didn't—and that maybe you didn't—in how powerful social networking can be. The good news is that you don't have to be a genius to master its potential.

Speak to your Colleagues:

Speaking, lecturing, and writing from your position of expertise is a great way to promote yourself and build your reputation. If there is any opportunity for you to get in front of other professions, be it in healthcare, fitness, or anything related, you should seize that chance. As a rule, people will only do business with the ones that they like, the ones that they trust, and the ones that they know. If you can get in front of people so they actually meet with you and vibe with you, you've created a great starting point. Maybe they'll like your personality and your demeanor; it could be as superficial as liking the way you look, but it all makes a huge difference in whether they'll do business with you or not.

Having these meetings, speaking in front of groups, and networking your own personality as a result of these opportunities is something you should never hesitate to do personally. It falls squarely in your top 5%, if you refer to the 95-5 Rule. And to get the chance to do this, you have to make your opportunities happen. You might write up a letter beforehand. In marketing space we would probably technically call it a sales letter. But in the healthcare space I'd prefer to call it an "introduction letter" or a "value proposition." In it, you're basically just telling the other healthcare provider how you can help them, what value you can bring to their services, or how you can make their services even better.

That letter is the best thing to start with, and then after you send it, you might want to follow up with an e-mail. Then finally, stop by for an actual visit, and have a chat with the person you've been writing to. Or have a cup of coffee with them. Follow up is the key, though. People are busy, and that can be the biggest challenge.

The Follow-Up:

The follow-up is probably the most important part of networking—and of marketing in general—that most marketers and clinicians tend to forget. I'm writing about it here because it's a great way to tie your networking skills into your whole marketing plan.

Say you sent out a mailing for referrals. A lot of practice owners I know would sit back, proud of having sent out such a great piece, and wait for the floodgates to open. But they forget the benefits that could be reached by simply following up on it.

If you send out a video or a message to fellow clinicians, have a call go out a little while later asking, "Did Dr. Jenkins watch the video? What did she think?" Even if Dr. Jenkins never watched the video, what you've just done is still part of marketing and building a presence. Do something outside the box or tied to a time of year and follow up on it, and you can help establish yourself as someone memorable and willing to do something interesting. Often that's all you need.

Let me give you an example that works because it's outrageous. Most people I know have been sent by someone or other they know a certain online video from a site called JibJab. It comes around Christmastime, and they superimpose your face onto the head of a cute, dancing elf. These videos are available for just about every other holiday as well. Last year we did one for St Patrick's day with my entire staff's heads on the characters. You can send it out when looking for referral and at the end have the message, "Send me your patients!"

It comes with a catchy song, it's on a free site, and you can send it as a link in a letter that you can write up however you want. Then you can track the link to see how many people watch it—and use that to tailor your follow up.

Now, I don't want you as a clinician to do this. Your staff will make it much more fun than you would, so have one of your front desk assistants put it together; that's what the 95-5 rule teaches us.

Associations

I want briefly to bring up a potentially slightly touchy subject, but it's one that people have recently been asking me. If you're a physical therapist like me, no doubt you will be familiar with APTA, or the American Physical Therapy Association. If you're not a physical therapist, I'm willing to bet there's a similar organization that exists for your specialization.

Of course, being in APTA or an organization like it has a lot of networking benefits. As you might imagine, there are a lot of physical therapists who feel that APTA is not doing as much as it should be, and there are others who strongly support it.

Here's my view. Years ago, when I was a physical therapist working for someone else, I had to pay the APTA fees. And honestly, I found them to be pretty high. It was probably an entire paycheck for me to pay the yearly membership fee. Like many people, I paid it right after college, as it was seen as the thing to do right after graduation.

So students ask me about APTA all the time. They see the cost, and they want to know if they would be making a good purchase by paying that fee. What I tell them is always the same: "You pay for what you get, and you have to take advantage of it."

APTA and associations like it have the potential to be big resources if you take advantage of them, and at the time I didn't take advantage of APTA the way I could have. In the field of physical therapy, it's a controversial question, and it's about 50/50 or 60/40 as to whether my colleagues think the organization is doing enough. But on an individual level, it will be up to you to decide if you think you would take advantage of their services enough to justify the cost.

I can tell you one thing that your professional organization won't do: solve all your problems. It's probably fair to say that a lot of people are so disappointed with their professional organizations because they expect them to be universal cure-alls.

To practitioners making this kind of complaint, I always repeat that old adage: "If you're not part of the solution, you're part of the problem."

Quite frankly, I think a lot of people complain about things that don't make a difference in the final equation. Our time is better spent trying to find ways of solving these problems than complaining about them.

Too many private practitioners I meet rely on APTA and organizations like it to do their marketing, and I think that's a complete mistake. In my opinion, since marketing or business education is not provided, a vast majority of practice owners do not know how to properly promote their practice.

Running a national campaign means spending months on building a brand. It's simply not going to help your practice right off the bat. It doesn't have an exact—or even an approximate—connection to your local office and your personal niche, and that's what I have to try to explain to my practitioner clients all the time.

Chapter Nine

Promoting Your Practice

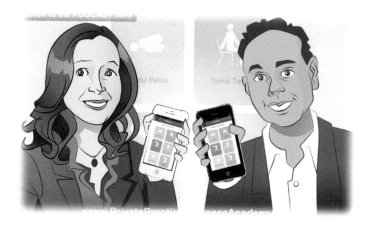

"If you're not embarrassed by the first version of your

product, you've launched too late."

– Reid Hoffman, co-founder of LinkedIn.

One of my biggest tasks in all the consulting I've done has been in speaking to established practitioners about the new generation of patients. Many people today find all their information online. That means that if they find you, it will have to be online, and if you portray your expert status to them at all, it will have to be online. If you are married to a marketing strategy from before the rise of the internet, you will soon be ignoring most of your potential clients.

If you are an established practice that already has an internet presence but is just starting to take advantage of the wave of the Medpreneur, there's a good chance you may need to buckle down and change your online persona. If you've had a website for years, you may need to make it more user friendly, or remove a lot of medical jargon to make it more approachable.

Look around you. The average person is now stuck to their phone—and that cell phone is everything for then. For a lot of people, the first reaction to feeling that they have a medical problem is not going to the doctor; it's trying to find their own diagnoses and treatments using their phone.

Using the internet and mobile phones isn't just generational. My father is in his seventies, and when he needs to find a plumber, he does it on his cell phone or tablet. You can't say that just because you have a geriatric population, you can ignore the necessity of being online. I often meet with coaching clients who tell me, "My client base just doesn't use the internet." Well, that may be—and if it is, it's important demographic information to bear in mind. But it certainly doesn't mean you can ignore the possibility of obtaining future clients through the internet, which will probably be their main way of finding you.

Start off with a Website

Maybe you already have a website. I worked with a doctor named Bill Lamberti, and he had one already too. But there was a problem; it was terrible. I couldn't believe it when I saw it. Now, let me disclaim this a little. I'm not actually a huge fan of overly ostentatious websites. If the website converts—if it's drawing in clients—it has done its job. Sometimes too many animations and too much elaborate coding can be counterproductive, and feel distracting for a potential client who just wants to log on and get good, straightforward healthcare information.

I have many business partners to this day who will fight me on the fact that they want a website to look pretty. I always say it's better to let the numbers speak for themselves. We sometimes even set up two sites for comparison, and we can track how many people come in from one site and how many come in from the other.

But I told Bill his website had to go. It was difficult to navigate, for one thing. It also lacked a call to action—that essential part of a pitch where a person is at last *told what to do:* to come to your practice. His site made no use of its prime real estate. In a website, prime real estate equates to the area "above the fold," which is to say the part of the site that is immediately visible in a viewer's browser before they scroll down at all. On Bill's site, the above the fold area was taken up entirely by a large photo that didn't tell me anything.

I told him, "When I go to your site, I have no idea whose site this is. I have no idea what services you actually provide." Most people decide whether to stay on a webpage in less than a minute, and a big picture with no information isn't going to convince them to do so. That's a lesson that's very simple but a lot of people still haven't learned, and it applies to all forms of advertising you might employ: people have to know what you're selling. Never get so creative with your PR that you lose the essential message.

When I gave Bill the feedback about his website, he had a very common reaction to critical feedback: his pride kicked in. "People are calling," he told me, "so obviously the website must be working."

It wasn't hard to rebut that. If the website was doing everything it should, why had he called me? We decided to go back to the site again and test it. And that's something you need to be able to do too. Let the numbers speak for themselves. We set up two sites and rotated them every two weeks or five-hundred views, whichever came sooner. As it happened, the new site converted 47% better, resulting in an average of two new patients per day. That is what I call a successful test.

Steps to a Great Website

It sounds like a simple question—what are the main features that work in a website? Naturally, you want it to be easy to navigate and easy to use. But how do you achieve that?

The first misconception to dispel about a great website is that you have to spend a lot of money on it. That's something a lot of people believe, but it simply isn't true. Your main goal is for your site to be functional, and functional websites these days are not expensive. The number of qualified web designers out there on the market has made the process of getting a website designed for yourself one that's actually very cheap.

How do you cut that cost, then? Are there so many web designers because it's so easy? I imagine a lot of people reading this might be wondering if they can simply make the site themselves. The answer is yes—but don't. It's like asking, "Can I go work out by myself?" Of course the answer is yes, but if you've never worked out before and you have no idea what you're doing, it is a good idea if you take somebody with you or hire a trainer.

If you're absolutely just starting and you can't budget anything for a site, you can create a WordPress blog and get online, because having that presence is essential. When considering time, efficiency, and expertise, you'll want to go to a professional who knows what they are doing and can deliver what you want. Don't go hire the number-one guy in the world—he's going to charge you a ton of money. Start by asking around and looking at other sites that you like.

Once you've got three or so sites you know you like from a user's perspective, you have something you can take to a web designer. If you know someone who does it, don't feel hesitant to give them the business; people are generally happy to send business back to someone who has given them business. It sounds like karma, but it's just a rule of how people work in doing business.

If you don't happen to know someone, don't hesitate to go to oDesk or Elance and list a job. Simply put, www.odesk.com and www.elance.com are sites that offer a service I've found really useful. Freelancers in any area can view your listing, and put in a bid on the service to be performed.

In this case, your order is going to be a simple one that, in terms of web design jobs, will be a fast and inexpensive one. You just need a one-page site. A one-page website with all the necessary information on it will do the job you want because, simply, that is where people start. The beauty of a website is that you can always add to it and grow it with more information and testimonials. As time goes on and you settle more comfortably into a niche, you'll be able to brand yourself with that Specialty. You'll also have more and data on who your clients are and what they are coming in for. You can use all of that to add to your website, but by no means does the site have to be massive right out of the gate.

What you *do* need to have on a website is what people are looking for when they look you up online. Clearly visible on your site and above the fold should be your contact information (address, telephone, and e-mail at least). It might feel strange to highlight these other methods of communication as part of your online presence, but just think how often you've searched through somebody's website trying to find out how to find them or call them on the phone.

Next, you need a strong headline of what it is exactly that you do. If you're a dentist, explain what style of dentistry you specialize in. In essence, what is the number-one thing that you are known for? You want the blurb version of your elevator pitch to be visible on your website. Never assume that people navigated there because they already knew exactly what they wanted.

Let people know they've reached the correct site. Are you the specialist located near their home or work? If someone quickly sees that the answer is yes, that's a huge plus for you. Make it easy for them to find you, because the less work they have to do, the easier it is for them to come to you. If you can include a map image or a link to how to get to your office on Google Maps, you've just increased your chances again.

You can't go wrong if you make it easy for them to find you, and you make it easy for them to call you. Then they'll call you to ask you any other questions they have, and once they're on the phone with you, that personal contact means that the ball is in your court and you already have the advantage.

On the one hand, the real point of the website is to get your name out there, and if it's done that, it has done its job. On the other, feedback can always help create a more pleasant experience. Personally, I update and clean up my website once or twice a year usually.

So don't fall in love with the first thing you have, and don't worry too much about the first version of your site, either. You'll always be able to change things to improve and fine tune them. By now, you might have thought of dozens of things to add to your site other than the ones I've mentioned—and that's fine. What I've recommended are the true essentials, and more can always be added as your site improves.

Video:

You do want to have a relevant picture, or if possible, a video. I'm big on videos because it turns out a lot of people do take the time to watch them when you feature them on the site. Any time they spend watching the video is time that you're making an impression on them, making it more likely that your name will stick with them when they're looking for a specialist.

133

Having a video humanizes you as well. If a potential client can click on a clip and see you speaking to them, they know *that's* who they're going to be dealing with when they come in and will immediately feel more comfortable. Fear most often grows out of uncertainty, and by showing yourself on film, you are peeling away a layer of uncertainty that people will have about your practice. Think about some local television ads you remember well; the fact that you recognize and feel like you know that guy from a hardware store down the street is a big asset to his business, even if he looks or sounds funny. So your first video should be about you. Introduce people, and show them who their doctor is.

Including a video has another huge advantage, which will help you keep your website down to that one page I suggested. If you can fit everything a client might need to know about your practice into a two-minute video (let's say), it will be more memorable, and it will also take up very little space on the website itself.

It's a huge asset if you can keep the site spare and still deliver all that information through the video. Plus, in a video clip, you control the running time, so you can spend as much time as you want highlighting what people should pay attention to.

One important lesson about the website that might seem a little counterintuitive: avoid talking about yourself too much. Instead, you want to give testimonials. These can be written, and they can definitely include pictures. But video testimonials work the best, because they have that personal connection I mentioned. Informational videos work really well, too, once you've established videos as something you do. In videos, as always, don't be scared of giving out information. It helps people, makes them like you, and establishes your credibility.

Most likely, you'll end up hosting your video on a site such as YouTube, and since Google now owns YouTube, video content gets a huge boost in Google search results. That's a big plus for you. You can augment your SEO by making sure to tag the video when you upload it so it gets picked up by the engine in more searches.

Making a short video is something fairly easy which virtually everyone can do, especially if you incorporate a PowerPoint presentation, which is a great way to incorporate a lot of information and simplify the production process.

There are apps you can use to make your own videos with smartphones; maybe you don't need to take advantage of that if you already have a camera. But my usual rule applies—if it's not efficient to do it yourself, outsource. There are plenty of video students and young filmmakers out there will take your commission. And once you have the finished product, a video doesn't have to just sit on your website but can be embedded in most of your social media sites to further help promote your practice. And as we learned above, if you can't do it, you can feel comfortable outsourcing it.

Now, I know right away what a lot of you are thinking right now. If you're brand new and you're just starting out, where are you going to get video testimonials? Well, you're absolutely right. You probably won't have video testimonials. Work with written testimonials for now, then work in video testimonials as they become available to you. That's just another way your presence can grow.

Share What You Know:

When people look for information these days, they look online. The practitioners they see there, they come to see as experts. As many have rightly pointed out, not all information on the internet is true. So I urge you: if you don't have an online presence yet, please get one as soon as possible, so you can build the expert reputation that you need and counter those who may be putting incorrect information out there.

To make an impact online, you have to follow a simple rule (and one which applies just as well offline too): give out as much free information as you can. This tends to frighten people when I say it.

People don't want to give away their best stuff. But I say, "That's what you should be doing. *Give away your best stuff!* People will want to come to you more because they think you have better stuff!"

Making this bold step is a real key to an effective presence. Sometimes I meet with multiple practitioners, and I always ask them to come up with the best idea they can and announce it to the whole room. Nobody wants to, because they are afraid others will now have the idea. They will—but more importantly they'll be convinced that the person who thought of it is pretty darn smart. A reputation like that is better than any one idea; it means people will want to come to you and ask you more questions. And that means clients.

136

Patients will always want to go to the person with the most knowledge. One of your important skills will be to take what you learned in medical school, or in journals, and repackage it so it's interesting, useful, and comprehensible for members of your client base.

Have a Mobile Presence:
I believe that mobile sites are a huge part of how people are finding practices today, and they're only going to get bigger. It's not something you can ignore. The fact that so many of us are as tied as we are to our phones means our first impressions of important websites will be via a mobile platform. That in mind, the clinician who didn't try to have a site that was at least compatible with mobile devices would be making a big error. That's something you can require of your web designer when assigning the work.

By a mobile site, I don't just mean one of those that will shrink down to the size of a cell phone's screen and be basically useable. You should have a separate mobile site that's different from the one that you already have. I have found that mine is especially useful, because with a mobile site you can include a call to action with a "call now" button right there.

Often someone who is late for an appointment will just Google your specialty while on their way. That person just needs your phone number. The best thing we added for our website was a button that says, "Running late? Call now!" That has banked us many new clients, and we've had many people directly thank us for it, too.

So every time I talk to a practice owner who doesn't have a mobile site, I try to direct them to a mobile website company. All the same design principles apply as on a desktop site, but you need to have one there because so many people are accessing the internet through cell phones these days.

Creating a Web Presence

So you've created your fantastic one-page website. Obviously, you want people to see it, and you want to put it everywhere. What's the best way to do that?

For starters, make sure that the website is attached to everything you do personally. Make sure it's on the signature of your e-mail. Put it on your business card and your stationery. Put it up in your practice. These are common strategies, but they're not everything.

You also want to make sure that your website gets publicized through social media and other high-traffic sites. This is part of a wider need for a web presence on the whole, which will be absolutely essential for you. Most practitioners I know have some vague idea about this, but no drive to implement it. They have accounts on most social networks, but they never post anything and have no content on their profiles. This helps nobody.

In fact, I think creating your web presence is one of the simplest but most effective things you can do in starting your practice. It's possible you've been reading this book so far with a little bit of wistfulness, because you don't have the spare cash yet to rent or lease out a space. That's fine. What you do have now is some free time. Remember, you're working nine to five still, and as soon as you're done, you have that time.

Remember how my wife started getting calls for appointments before she had a space, just because we started building her web presence? What you can do is start blogging, start a Facebook page, and generally start creating an expert reputation for yourself. If you put it out there, the community can find it and start asking for you. So even if you're still at square zero, your online presence can be a great way to generate that first client for you. It will never lose that level of importance, no matter how big your practice gets.

I already mentioned that Google Maps is a great way to help direct customers to your office, but that's far from the end of its usefulness. The first and most important step is getting your business listed on Google Maps. Many people use Google's business-place listings to find real businesses in their area, and determine the hours, directions, and contact information. In short, you want to show up on that map when people search Google for what you are. This step is free. Google is more than happy to put that up for you, because the more businesses they have listed, the more it helps their business model. So by not being on there, you would really be missing out. Google Maps is basically a way to start out with a freebee homerun for your practice.

Next, you want to leverage Facebook. Create a fan page, and even start talking up your practice on the personal Facebook page that you may already have. The message is simple. Something like, "Hey everyone. I just started my own practice, specializing in [your

139

specialty]. Check out my new website at [your website]. Please share this around to family and friends who might be interested."

Now, this isn't crass advertising. Remember, these are your friends on Facebook you're sharing this with. Pretty universally, people are going to be happy for you and proud of you. They're absolutely going to look at your site, because as your friends, they're automatically interested. If they think it's ugly or they don't like it for some other reason, that's still great. Take the feedback. They're your test audience, and you can use them to help find out how strangers will react.

Not just on Facebook, your own social media is the way to start. This is where to find "low-hanging fruit," so to speak, because the people there already like you and trust you. When they start referring their own friends and family, it's the best kind of word of mouth. And when you start getting video testimonials from them, you can see how everything starts to come together and the ball really starts rolling. When you're just starting out, test the waters. Spending thousands on Google AdWords or an ad in a magazine isn't something you're ready for . . . yet.

You'll get reviews on your Google Maps, page, and on review sites such as Yelp. You should pay attention to these, since they legitimately affect how many customers make their choice today, but because the content is user-generated, the responses can be unpredictable and sometimes untruthful.

Now, I have a lot of dental clients, for instance, who have told me they absolutely despise Yelp, because it allows people to post inaccurate, untruthful reviews. That's true. You'll get good reviews, and you'll get bad reviews; you just have to learn how to roll with it. I myself have had a bad review, and that's just what I did.

I think, to a certain extent, it actually helps the patient see that no one is perfect. One bad review among a set of mostly good ones can actually help to humanize you. There's no reason you can't address those bad reviews. Turn them into opportunities and respond. Explain what you're doing to solve the problem that's been brought up. That takes a lot of courage because it involves addressing your enemies, but it can turn a bad situation into a good one.

On the whole, you should concentrate on the good rather than the bad. Go to those patients who were highly satisfied; ask them for good reviews or for referrals. You have the greatest possible advantage there: they like you already. Bad reviews eat at a practitioner, because you want to be the best you can be to everyone. One I got certainly eats at me. But one or two negative comments over the course of a years-long career actually means you're doing very well, considering that, in this world, you just can't help everybody all the time.

We don't live in a perfect world, and unfortunately, you may have the experience of a competitor going onto your site and posting bad reviews. A site like Yelp doesn't have the means or technology to detect these posts and remove them. It's something that just has to be dealt with. It doesn't mean you should throw in the towel on encouraging online reviews, because if you don't have enough or you have too many bad ones, it can palpably hurt your business.

Blogging

Here's a rule that's always true, and especially true when you're starting out: good marketing content is informative. The way to get people to pay attention to your marketing material is shockingly simple; you want to put out great content and educational pieces. As a healthcare practice, you're built for that. You already have a wealth of great information the public largely doesn't know about.

If you're a podiatrist, you probably know some simple ways to relieve common sources of foot pain. Put that simple information out there somehow, and you will be surprised at how many people respond to that and see a real benefit from it. Down the road when they have more foot problems, or when they need to refer a friend, they can contact you directly through your page, and you've got a new private.

I've mentioned already that blogging is a great way of getting online and starting a web presence for yourself. You may already have made the connection that blogs are ideal ways of getting content and information out to a widespread public, spreading the awareness and credibility of your practice.

Blogs have a high level of public awareness, with frequent mentions of "the Blogosphere" on the news, and a lot of practitioners come to me asking whether I think they should start a blog. Beyond having the word *blog* in their head, they have no further idea of where to start.

There are a lot of ways to get your blog online, and probably the best one to go with if you're starting out is WordPress, which is a very versatile, user-friendly, and free online service. If you want greater control over your content, you can also go with a self-hosted blog, which any web designer you hire should be able to build into the design of your site for you.

Your blog can be very important, because along with your site it represents the only "real estate" you have online. It's your voice on the internet, and you own that. If you have strong opinions to express and good information to disseminate, blogs are the way to do that in a way that stays online and is under your own banner, rather than that of Facebook or some other site.

But what to do write on your blog? Well, an important thing to remember is the etymology. Blog is simply short for web log, and that's what it is. It's not a set of unrelated informational articles on various subjects. Those are great, but they're best kept on your main site where they can be accessed for information and indexed without being tied to a particular moment in time.

While a blog is a great way for you to educate and inform people, it is also a vehicle for you to create a personal identity and reputation online. That can lead to confidence and exposure among potential clients. People tend to trust people more when they already know who they are, and even more so if they've somehow been helped by them. Now, blogs tend to come up a lot for me when my clients bring up what they can have their staff do to help improve the practice. It's natural that people should be interested in this; if you're paying staff, you want to be able to get the most that you possibly can out of them.

I certainly know a few people who are asking their employees to write their blogs for them. Is this effective? It could be. The numbers aren't out yet, and as far as I know, not a lot of people are even tracking it in the first place. If you couldn't tell already, I'm very big into tracking numbers and analytics on everything I do for my practice.

I'm proud of that because I think it's the correct way to proceed. But there are a lot of practitioners out there playing staff to blog for them while they're just not doing anything to track where their referral sources are actually coming from. See whose posts get the most hits or cause the most referrals, and keep those writers blogging.

Whether you or your staff does it, it's important to blog on a regular basis. I know people who start a blog, put one up, and don't come back to it for three or four months. It doesn't matter if you write every week, every other week, or what. But it helps to have a consistent schedule so people come back consistently. And if you've succeeded in your goal of providing good information that people are interested in, it will create a sense of anticipation.

As we've mentioned, there's no cost to starting a blog. So at the beginning there's no risk. But if you put a lot of effort and time in with no reward there is; the old adage that "time is money" is a true one. Having an employee start a blog brings a lot of value to the practice, but you want to make sure to track those numbers.

If you're seeing a benefit, you absolutely continue with it. If you have different employees writing different posts, you want to track whose posts get the most hits and whose posts get the most comments.

Chapter Ten

Marketing Magic: Advertising

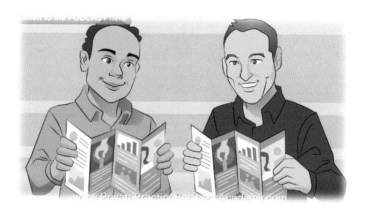

"Genius is 1% inspiration, and 99% perspiration."

– Thomas Edison

Advertising and marketing are by no means the same thing, but advertising can and should be a big part of marketing. And I want to say right to most physicians, dentists, physical therapists, and other health and wellness providers one thing: your advertising sucks.

It sucks because so much of health and medical advertising just does the same thing. We spend most of the time in our ads just talking about how good we are. It might seem a little counterintuitive, but that's really not what we need to do.

In my estimation, an advertisement that just says, in essence, "I am the best at this," is only going to work about 20% of the time. If you're happy with that, that's fine. But know that your competition is out there, and they're advertising better every day.

The number one thing to remember about advertising is this: if you advertise like everyone else, you're going to get everyone else's results. That is just absolutely unsatisfactory. Do not copy your competitor's advertisement, then come back and say that print, website, or direct mail advertising doesn't work. All that means is that it didn't work for you. In this section, I'm going to go through a host of potential advertising methods to bring clients through your door. Don't dismiss any, because the most effective practices usually use multiple strategies at once.

Print and the Advertorial

Print is usually the most standard form of advertising people think of, and by no means is it dead. Print advertising is fantastically effective in a lot of cases, but you absolutely have to know your target audience. Let me start with an example.

I just talked with a client of mine down in Baltimore who does dry needling, which is a form of acupuncture. She asked if I could create an ad for her. I'm not an ad writer per se, but I've done enough copywriting and created enough advertisements that I know what will work. In that area, I'm pretty knowledgeable, because I myself have done dry needling as a physical therapist.

So I charged her an appropriate fee since I was going outside of my normal services, and we sat down to put an advertisement together. I told her I couldn't promise anything; there were simply too many variables. I could get people to call her clinic, but if the front desk staff couldn't schedule them or get them to actually come in through the door, or if she couldn't sell them on cash-based services, then she wouldn't make money. In that circumstance, the ad didn't fail, but her staff failed.

In general, a print ad works so well that I could put one out for you and flood your clinic with phone calls. But if your staff drops the ball on converting sales, you still lose money. Now, when I do this, I often even set up my own line attached to the number and have my own people answering the phones and accessing clients' schedules, just to eliminate that chance of error. That way I prove to them that it really works, and the power of advertising is not just make-believe.

For greatest effectiveness, I think a print ad should contain a story. After all, that's why people are reading a print medium in the first place. To my mind, the advertorial works better than anything. It's not as easy to get into a newspaper, but usually if you have a history with a newspaper and have run a few ads with them already, they might let you do one. That's just one place where you have to spend a little money to make a little money.

What is an advertorial? In its most basic form, it's a story. Take a look at *Men's Health*, or *Men's Fitness*, or any magazine like that. Flip through. Sooner or later, you'll see a story with a picture of a bulky-looking muscular guy, with some text about his pre-workout routine and how he builds muscle. If you keep reading, somewhere in there they start talking about whey protein, how it builds muscle, and how it has changed the way he gets ready to work out. If you read further, there's an offer asking you to send away for a free sample of whey protein.

By the time you're at the third page, you often don't realize you were reading an ad the entire time because you were so engrossed in the magazine. That concept works the same way for healthcare. Let's say we place an ad called *The Three Easy Ways to Cure Back pain.* We start by talking about how Mrs. Jones was shoveling snow, and she threw out her back. The neighbor had to come over and help her out; they went to the ER, etcetera.

By the time you've written all this, people have become engrossed in the story. In the middle of it, you can describe how the attending told Mrs. Jones to go to your particular physical therapy clinic, and now you're just talking about your own practice and how they didn't just give the standard service that everyone else would. By the time a reader is at the end of the page, they don't realize that they've been heavily pitched on the physical therapist.

So many people end up thinking, "I have a problem with that. I should go see a physical therapist. This guy's right in my home town, and they wrote a story about him." It doesn't matter that it was really just a giant ad. Done correctly, the advertorial is massively powerful because most people don't realize they're being sold anything—it's just the story coming through.

If you can augment the advertorial with someone backing your claim, that's even better. If the physician who tells Mrs. Jones to go to your clinic is a local doctor who will promote you, then you both get some light shed on your own services. That can also be a great joint venture where both practices work together to help absorb the cost of the advertorial.

Just last year, I ran that "Mrs Jones" advertorial, and I even paid the extra fee to run it all weekend. It ended up being a huge homerun for me, probably helped in part by the fact that we had such a bad winter around where I work!

But should you be writing about Mrs. Jones shoveling snow, or Judy spraining an ankle in her high school lacrosse game? You'll hear me say it a million times: you can't dismiss the importance of demographics. It's almost like peeling an onion to get to the very core of your client base. Then you'll know exactly who you're writing the story for, and the effect can only come then. Otherwise you're talking to the air.

Let me tell you about a couple sins that get committed in advertising all the time, which really undermine the intentions of the people who commit them.

The First Sin of Print Advertising:

The first Sin of Advertising is that of paying too much attention to your logo. The thing about sins is that it's very easy to succumb to the temptation to commit them, and this is no exception most of us think of a logo as something integral to an advertisement.

Dr. Joseph Simon

But let's think about in. In any advertisement, no matter what format or size it is in, the top 25% of space is the prime real estate. And in a lot of advertising I've seen, that top 25% is given to the logo. You might already have taken out an advertisement like that. Now, I use logos, too. There's nothing wrong with them, but they don't constitute advertisements in and of themselves.

Think about the advertisement you're putting out to your patient population. Here is my question: Is your brand really so strong that your logo itself commands people's attention and convinces people to become your clients?

Is the name of your practice the most important thing that could be said about your business? Is that name the most interesting and persuasive thing that could be said to a potential patient? If not, it should be at the bottom of your advertisement, not at the start.

The Second Sin of Print Advertising:

The second sin of advertising is omitting a headline. Removing your logo from its perch in the prime real estate of your ad does not mean that there should be nothing left there. There's almost no justification for an ad without a headline. I want your advertisement to scream, "Attention patients! Attention patients!" And never forget the power of specificity—if you do root canals you basically want it to say, "Attention, root canal patients!"

I want your advertisement to shout out to the exact pain that is felt by your particular demographic. That's what we're here for. Our task as healthcare providers is to talk about their pain. I want them to

150

swivel their head to see your advertisement and wonder what it is talking about. I want them to think, "Is this ad talking about me?"

Only then do I want them to see your logo or your name at the bottom of the advertisement and say, "Oh! I know them. That's the practice down the street." If they recognize you, that's great. If the logo helps them to do that, so much the better. But none of that is going to help unless you have a headline that grabs their attention.

The mistakes I'm telling you about are hard to avoid, and that is in no small part because they're also made by the majority of brand advertisers that you run into. If you just walk into a newspaper office and say that you want an advertisement, the person you talk to is likely just to give you something bog-standard, with a big logo and no headline.

But I've got to put it bluntly: that's dumb. It's simply stupid and wrong, but the person you're dealing with doesn't know any better than to give you this advice. I do know better, and I'm giving you better advice: you can't put out an advertisement without a headline if you want it to be successful.

How do you put that headline together? Like many things, it has to be tailored to your practice and your niche, but the universal element is that it has to catch attention. It has to be alarming, it has to be news, and it has to make some kind of promise.

That promise, of course, must be something to do with what your practice can do. Promise them how and why they will get better, show them proof, and offer them testimonials. Show Mr. Johnson, whom you treated recently. Maybe he lost forty pounds with

151

gastric bypass surgery or your special diet, or maybe you cured his hemorrhoids. But the important thing is to show his smiling face on the right side of the before-and-after graphic.

Testimonials tend to work fantastically well, because they appeal to our sense of trust and human interest in the patient. If you can get a testimonial from someone well-known or respected in your community, that's a huge bonus. And it grabs attention all on its own.

Let me give you a good example of how effective a striking image can be. I was working with a dentist not long ago, and we decided to go with an ugly teeth advertisement. We used one of his patients, omitting his full face and name. We just used a picture of his teeth. Our prime real estate just showed a big picture of his ugly teeth, above the headline, "Is this you?"

Let me tell you, we had more phone calls to the practice than I had ever seen, because so many people did not want to be this person. People immediately thought, "I'm not sure if it's me! I don't think I'm this bad." It commanded attention and then spurred them on into making the call and setting up an appointment.

That was something that worked fantastically, and there's one other thing there worth noting, by-the-by. Ugly teeth are ugly. That's fine. Your attention-grabber doesn't have to be something people would choose to look at; it has to be something that will get the job done and bring attention to your practice.

You don't need to use that piece of shiny, new equipment that you just bought, and in fact, I would rather you didn't. It's not dramatic, and it's not specific to your practice. So it won't set you apart from the pack.

Great advertising is memorable and personal. It may require you to think outside your familiar terms of reference. For example, years ago, somebody mentioned to me a personal theory that if you went out onto the street and asked a hundred people what they thought physical therapy was, only about four of them would be able to give you a real concrete answer.

That really struck me, and as soon as I heard it, I made a change. I stopped advertising, "physical therapy," and started advertising directly to people with pain of whatever type I wanted to target. I started saying, "back pain," or, "shoulder pain," in my advertising, and the response skyrocketed. It's still tough for me today when I see so many practices with advertising that just says, "physical therapy."

So get out there and start coming up with ideas for headlines. Write everything down that you come up with, no matter how crazy. Look back over what you've got, and you'll be able to see what grabs your attention most strongly. Whatever it is, that's what you've got to go with.

Billboards

You do have to be careful with ads you buy in general, for one simple reason. The person selling you the ad is trying to do just what you are: generate a sale. It's our job to make sure the deal is as beneficial to us as it is to them.

Billboards are not a method I've ever recommended to my clients. They're very expensive and tend to look like showboating, so I've never felt confident enough in their return on investment to feel comfortable recommending them.

The most important rule is always to do what works best for your own practice. In my home state of New Jersey, I see a bariatric center using a billboard on the New Jersey Turnpike what seems like every month. Over a couple years, I've never seen the ad come down. So I know the guy who put it up must either be getting a return or like throwing money out the window.

If you're financially secure enough for the expenditure, a risk like a billboard seems like the kind that could pay off big, or could pay nothing at all.

Cost of Advertising

When I talk to marketing clients, I often get the question, "How much would it cost for this kind of campaign?" When I give them a quote, the question tends to follow: "Will I get that money back right away?"

Not to lean too heavily on generalizations, it happens that a lot of these questioners tend to be physical therapists. When they are, or when they come from one of a good number of other fields that for many years didn't have to advertise heavily, I tell them one thing: look at dentists.

Dentists, in general, have learned over time to invest money in their marketing. They've absorbed the lesson that if you put one dollar in, you'll eventually get two dollars back. Sometimes that's a difficult concept to impress on a physical therapist or another practitioner who's been used to getting business only from physician referrals.

So I find myself telling people all the time, "Watch what your local dentist is doing." One patient doesn't leave a dentist and go to another; that whole patient's family comes along. When I coach dentists, they often immediately know where I'm going with the points I'm making about generating more referrals.

That's true because for years, it has been necessary for them to be attuned to the power of marketing their own practices. And that situation is slowly coming about for other specializations as well. A big shift is coming, and I've seen both older and newer practices start to take advantage of marketing. That will mean those who do not will be left behind. As I previously stated, a man once told P. T. Barnum that he couldn't afford to advertise. Barnum famously replied, "My friend, you can't afford not to advertise." I think that's already true in the healthcare field today, and it's getting truer all the time.

Of course, it doesn't mean that you shouldn't take note of the costs of various forms of advertising. Google advertisements are very cheap if you handle them right, and can be very effective because they allow you to target people by demographic. You can allot a hundred dollars to test out one advertisement, and just see what happens. Will Google pick it up? Will some other website pick it up? I don't know, but if one patient walks in through the door and spends a thousand dollars, that Google ad was more than enough.

Your costs are reduced when you only spend on what works. If you know how Google does for you, try placing a Facebook advertisement. Wherever it is, if you can target your advertising well enough that it works, you're probably not spending too much.

155

I like to do a little thought experiment with clients. I ask them, "What does one patient cost?" We sit down, and we do the math. We plot out what the value of that patient's one visit is, then we work out what their lifetime value would be if they come back over a couple of years. If for the sake of easy math, we say one visit is worth a hundred dollars, and a lifetime is worth a thousand, then my rule is that you have anywhere between a hundred and thousand dollars to spend on each sure patient you can pull in.

If it's a matter of bringing in someone brand new, I would say not to spend more than the hundred-dollar figure on a campaign or an ad. Your chances are lower with these people than with those who have already proven that they would come in at least once. Once you have a patient, you can start spending more money on that individual person.

If they're already drawing attention to themselves, raising their hand, and telling you what problem they have, you basically know they're going to come. So spending the money to ensure that is a sound investment. Then you can drop some real money on following that person around the internet with ads, because you know they already have an interest in what you provide.

I recently consulted with somebody whose one-time fee to see a patient was $750. And you can run a ton of ads on Facebook or Google for a sum like that. At my own practice I have to be careful to keep my numbers low, because I can only justify spending around forty-nine dollars on an individual new patient. Now, I want to make it clear: this is only the up-front cost. Once they are in my funnel, I can go up to $1,000 in advertising.

Your Budget for Marketing
Of course, the importance of the cost of advertising is going to be dependent on your overall budget for advertising. And overall, I find that the practice owners I encounter are less open than they should be to dedicating space in their budget to advertising.

As a very general rule, it's usually advisable to spend around 8-10% of the practice's budget on advertising. On average, owners tend to spend only around two and a half percent. What often happens is not that they immediately go under, but that they either see very limited, slow growth from it, or swing back and forth between good months and bad months because they're not willing to put the money in that they need to for strong, sustained growth.

That said, every practice is going to have some months that are better than others. I've seen plenty where there is a pattern in place. Many practices follow the school year and are very busy during the fall and spring, but basically dead during the summer and over the holiday season. At that point, practitioners often start panicking and looking for solutions because they don't know what they will do for the rest of the season.

I see it all the time, and when I go into a practice for the first time, there's no way of knowing what their patient-to-revenue ratio will be—let alone patient to employee. One way for people to use revenue in a way that can actually affect that ratio is to invest seriously in marketing.

If that describes your practice, you need to build for factors that you already know are in place. You prepare for the slow season and start marketing or setting up your marketing early, so you can keep the success of the practice steady.

It might be hard to fathom using up to 10% of your budget on marketing; it might seem like too big a chunk out of whatever number you're looking at, especially if you're just starting out. But it's not an expense you can ignore.

Educational Marketing

A lot of clinicians have relied on referrals and word-of-mouth for a long time. You know by now that I don't think that should be your only resource by any stretch of the imagination. However, the idea that you have no control over whether or not you get referrals or good word-of-mouth is a myth.

You can market for referrals through existing clients. Well-designed incentives for patients who refer friends and acquaintances can do wonders. Sometimes the simplicity of just providing an opportunity wins out. Statistically, people are much more likely to refer a friend if you provide them with some kind of form to do it with. So there's no reason not to hand these forms out at events and in the office, and to have a similar option on your website.

As always, providing information is great. Informative content is the kind that people pass on to their friends, as you can discover just by taking a look at your e-mail inbox. In an indirect way, we're using our own patients to help us, and encouraging word of mouth when we direct them to this good content. There's no reason to not do this, or encourage them proactively to tell their friends, "Give us a good review on Yelp, or do any number of things that can help spread awareness about our practices."

Chapter Eleven

Beyond the Practice: Selling Your Services

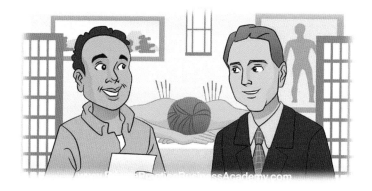

"Logic will get you from A to B. Imagination will take

you everywhere."

– *Albert Einstein*

Developing a Product

Thinking about your practice as a product you're selling, can be just as beneficial as thinking of it as a traditional clinic. If you have the opportunity, you can use the development of an actual product as a great way to generate revenue as well as to promote your practice.

161

Needless to say, having another revenue stream means you can invest back into your practice and continue to improve.

In a lot of cases, it has been helpful to people to develop a product that has a recurring revenue factor built into it. If you have the kind of practice where it's appropriate, you may consider selling supplements, for instance. While you may start by taking a loss on the pills themselves, you can build them into a program that over time will both make you money and encourage your patients to remain repeat clients. If you get people into a program where you're guaranteeing their participation for six months, you've gifted yourself with a great compliance factor.

There are a lot of people out there who want to do this, but have been budgeting themselves carefully and may not have the funds to develop it at the outset. That's why I recommend starting development very simply. When a product is involved you can start to get involved with crowdfunding. Services like IndieGoGo and Kickstarter will allow you to raise money for the public to develop of your products; you just need to come up with creative prizes for your public that donors will receive at different cash levels. Kickstarter requires you to set a dollar-amount goal and doesn't pay you if you don't reach it, so IndieGoGo is a less risky proposition. The response level you get can be a great litmus test of how the public responds to your products. It's the broader, modern equivalent of, say, going to an angel investor for money for a new piece of equipment for your clinic.

My main piece of advice with regard to creating a product is this: you don't have to be an inventor to have an invention. All you have to do to is "remix" or combine some existing ideas in a useful way. There a million products out there, and the key to easily developing something of your own is to take something out there and make it somehow better or easier. You can combine two things that are already out there to make something of your own.

Of course, your main question has to be, "Will people pay for this?" Don't go right out and dump a fortune on a prototype or a patent lawyer. If you can make a makeshift model by taping or stapling a few things together, please do that instead. Make it really cheap, and then test it out in your own clinic. That's the best way to see if it's even worth the time and effort to create a prototype or buy a patent, because it costs you nothing.

What most people do not know is that submitting a provisional patent costs only $97, and you can do it online. That gives you a whole year to promote the product, sell it, and even license it out to a bigger company. After that year you can either go ahead with a full patent, or you can ditch the product altogether and move on to something new.

After you have your provisional patent, move onto a makeshift prototype that you can show people and test out yourself. Use that to test the product and make sure it really works. See whether people like it, and whether they will pre-order the product. Say to them, "This is going to be coming out in a few months. Do you want to order it now?"

If people actually put money down on a product, that's how I know I have a winner. And as soon as I know I have a winner, I start pitching that product to bigger companies and trying to license it out. I personally don't want to manufacture and sell it; I'd rather just make the money and sell units.

In my case, I most recently partnered up with somebody to develop a piece of exercise equipment we call the Stability Lock. It's a long, clear cylinder with handles, and you can lift it over your head, do bench presses with it, and more. The takeaway is that the product has water inside, so it causes an instability when you carry it.

All my partner and I did was combine two products together and add handles. I know a lot of readers are saying to themselves at this point, "I've seen this concept before!" Exactly. You've seen the concept before, but we've changed it. All we had to do was change one very small feature of it.

Marketing Your Product - Barry Khan's 110% Play Harder

I don't want to pick on podiatrists in particular, but it seems like every time I go into a podiatry practice, they have orthotics sitting out for sale. Invariably, they just keep sitting there and don't get sold. Needless to say, they're doing nobody any good. You need to have a way to sell a product if you have it.

That should proceed naturally. Patients want their healthcare provider to take care of them. So if you believe in what you're selling and present it as something that will help the patient's treatment, you are perfectly positioned. If you believe in it, the patient will too. That's better than selling. And it's truly showing your value.

As with the marketing of anything, finding and creatively exploiting a niche is still your number one priority. I talked, for instance with Barry Khan, Director of Clinical Business at 110% Play Harder (http://www.110playharder.com). Barry's company was founded with the specific mission of helping athletes recover quickly and soundly from playing hard, particularly with the idea of helping endurance athletes, such as marathon runners, triathletes, and long distance runners.

Now, that's niching down right from the start, and his firm knew that they could take advantage of their body of patients even more strongly if they introduced a product. What they chose to sell goes to prove that to reap great advantages just from the introduction of a product to a practice, you don't have to be an inventor, and you don't have to bring in anything needlessly complicated.

At its most basic, the product is a compression sleeve with ice packets built in. David Green, the president of the company acquired the product and introduced it, making sure to emphasize that its design allowed for an unprecedented level of comfort in compression, due to a two-layer design and specially-designed soft fabric.

It's a simple, inexpensive design with a practical use. I know from experience, that often if you give young athletes a traditional ice pack, they'll put it on while playing a video game, then not bother to hold it on once it falls off. So the product of Barry's firm could ensure compliance in that area by 100%, as I see it, because the pack is wearable. This underscores an important point: your product has to serve a legitimate, useful purpose. You don't want to scam people, and you're not a bar where people will want to wear your name on a T-shirt.

As Barry told me about his product, "Every single clinic owner I talk to and present our product to has said, 'Yes. I would like to have that available to my patients.'"

Now, that seems miraculous, but these things are possible when you fit neatly into a niche. There are niches for selling to other clinic owners just as there are for attracting clients. I don't need to tell you what a fantastic source of revenue it could be to have sales coming in from your own clients alongside ones from other practices.

I asked Barry to explain a bit about how he makes it work. He told me, "Here's why I'm getting 100% acceptance. The barriers to turning the clinical space into a retail space have traditionally been upfront costs, inventory storage, and the actual cost in space of the place to see the products in the clinics. A lot of therapists don't have the time or money to set up a retail store within their clinics. So what we decided to do was to set up a non-stock retail platform for the clinic space. The only upfront expense is a marketing kit. It comes like a full run of samples, a prescription pad, a functioning site, and some official marketing literature. That's it. That's all. We route all the orders through the portal and deliver straight to the patient's home."

The practice essentially operates as an online retailer from the venue of the office. This makes it very easy for the clinic to generate a brand new revenue stream, and at the same time to give their employees what in effect can be a new kind of incentive. If you give them an incentive, the employees can, in a certain measure, be in charge of their own destinies as far as generating extra income for themselves.

It's the best of both worlds. I used to sell products in my own practice, and I would have loved to take advantage of a way not to have to reorder supplies every so often and find a place to store them. But you don't want to lose the advantage of an in-person sale. You can have somebody at the clinic mention something and hope the patient will go home later and buy it, but there's always going to be a turnaround time that will give interest a chance to wane. If you're selling in the office, you can simply work with a greater confidence rate that the patient will buy.

This is where skill in building a team plays in again as well. As I'm sure you can tell by this point, all elements of running your practice are really interconnected. A lot of clinic owners have difficulty selling in the first place, and your average therapist or doctor is just not going to do it out of the blue.

It can help to have somebody trained on staff to know—and know how to sell—your product. That can be somebody who can show the product as a legitimate piece of medical equipment, try it on the patient, show them how it works, then hand the patient off to an associate to walk them through purchasing it on the website.

Success Story - Jeff Worrell

For my podcast, I recently interviewed Jeff Worrell, the VP of the company Rehab Division, which provides supplies to the physical therapy, message, and chiropractic industries. He's also the host of another popular podcast related to our profession, **PT Talker**, which has been on the air for about six years. Jeff's been in the physical therapy business since 1986, after training as an athletic trainer in college. He helped bring to market what was then a revolutionary prophylactic knee brace for football players. He saw his opportunity, and within two years, started his own physical therapy supplies firm. Jeff has some great advice about selling, and it starts with an unorthodox rule: "I don't sell anything."

As he explains, "If I am a patient, and my healthcare professional believes that there is a product or service that would assist me in having a better outcome, I actually want them to introduce me to it, tell me about it, and make sure I'm aware. It then becomes my decision as the patient whether or not I want turn over the dollars for that. I don't look at it as selling. I advise clients who struggle with retail opportunities, and I tell them, 'You're not selling. You're providing additional services.' The bottom line is that you wouldn't have it in your office if you didn't honestly believe that there was value and benefit to your patients. Patients do not want to go to K Mart or Target to find a product; they want their healthcare provider to take care of them. This should be a natural extension!"

And that philosophy, in my opinion, is better than selling. It transcends a simple pitch if you really believe in what you are showing your customers. If you believe in it, your patient is going to believe in it.

Jeff sees his industry as changing, and focusing in recent years more on an entire wellness approach than on fixing one individual problem or another. That leads to a shift in the client psyche towards smaller, more conservative, and less specialized equipment being bought. "But," he says, "I advise my clients not to get so generic with their equipment that they look like the Gold's Gym next door. Obviously the patient is coming to physical therapy for something very different than what they want from Gold's Gym. You want to make sure the equipment has a medical feature to it that would be important to people who are dealing with an illness. On the whole, I like to offer my clients equipment that will do one of three things: offer a better patient outcome, save money, or save time."

And as for why he puts the work into his podcast that he does, Jeff offered me a simple explanation. "I'm out there trying to be of help to my clients. I want to help my industry. I want to provide expertise and information to clients. I started talking to them about just how they sort through all the information they're presented with every day, and it occurred to me that I could present an expert for ten minutes or so every week and build up a library of this information; it would stay relevant throughout the year. That's why I committed to the weekly podcast."

I've been on Jeff's show, and it was a great experience. There's a lot you'll be able to take away from it, whether you're a physical therapist yourself or not! For more from Jeff, take a listen to his appearance on my own podcast: http://privatepracticebusinessacademy.com/pttalkradio/

Chapter Twelve

Putting It All Together

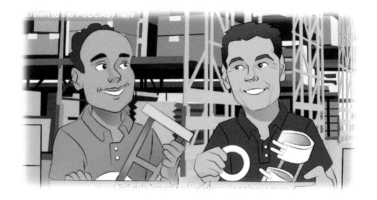

"No one wants physical therapy (or your service), but

they need physical therapy"

– Dr. Joe Simon

Once you have clients coming in, it's imperative to establish a base, and keep a good proportion of those clients coming back to you. Patient loyalty is one of the most important things you can secure for your practice. The biggest problem most practices have, whether they know it or not, is that they take advantage of a very low percentage of patient loyalty—often almost zero.

Most patients' experience is that they have one injury or illness, they go to their primary care doctor, and he or she either refers them out to a specialist or solves the problem right there—and that's it. The question we need to ask is this: If you treat a patient for, say, back pain, what is that patient going to do the next time he or she has back pain? Will they come back to you, or will they go on what they got based on word-of-mouth from a friend? Maybe they'll be a town over and will head to whichever doctor is nearest because making it back to your practice will be too far.

Missing that patient's business on a repeated basis means losing a huge opportunity. To take advantage of the potential of patient loyalty, you need a system in place that's planned and implemented. And for that, your staffing couldn't be more important. Everyone on staff—everyone from the receptionist to the administrative staff has to understand how the system works and how it is put into practice.

The patients themselves, in fact, have to be educated on the fact that we expect patient loyalty. You need to impress upon them explicitly the message that they shouldn't be going somewhere else—if they have a problem with what your practice treats, they should be coming to you. Even if they have another problem, they should still be coming to you, if only because they should trust you to know how best to refer them out correctly.

Make sure your staff knows—and implements—the policy that on a patient's first visit, they tell him or her you can take care of more than one issue. If the treating clinician mentions that to them, the average patient might say, "I just need to feel better." That's your goal, too. But whenever it is that they are feeling better, say after the fourth or fifth visit, that's when the administrative staff can pick up the message. Make sure they know to tell patients they can refer their friends, and that you're the go-to practice for your particular field.

The most important and effective way of making a message or a piece of information stick with someone is repetition. To make it stick even better, create an emotional connection with them as well. And that's why you need to make sure the message that reinforces loyalty is repeated to the patient at as many points and in as many contexts as possible. It may seem over-the-top to you, but it will mean that message is driven home, and patient will be much more likely to come back.

You also have to impress upon people the concept that they may need to come in even though they don't feel like there's anything wrong with them at a given moment. That will be counterintuitive to a lot of your clients, but it's very important.

For instance, among the practices I've visited, many were sports medicine and fitness-based. What we often see there is a huge number of muscle imbalances in the body of a so-called healthy individual. The patient can't feel them on his or her own, but they're there. Practitioners have tested therapies that work on these, and when the muscle imbalances are corrected, you can actually see the patient moving two, three, or even 4% faster.

It's true in every field that there are things you could do for a patient—things that would achieve the equivalent of that 4% gain in speed for them—even though they already feel happy and well. Our techniques have to reach that average member of the public who feels fine. We have to let that person know that just because you feel good right now doesn't mean that if you don't maintain it or don't exercise, you won't feel worse in the future. But how do you convince them of that?

Of course, eventually there will be arthritis or an ACL injury or something along those lines to deal with. In fourteen years, I've seen it occur time and time again. By fixing a muscle imbalance on one side we prevent an ankle sprain down the road on the other side. Doubtless you can think of equivalents of this phenomenon in your own specialty.

The Mindset Shift

I know it's not easy being out there in the struggle, because I've done it, and I still do it myself. I'm not just a marketer, and I'm not somebody out there peddling bad advice. I participate in every aspect of this business. So the strategies I've talked about—strategies to help grow your business and grow your marketing presence—are effective ones that I've worked through myself. And I'd go so far as to say that they're a necessity.

There's a lot of advice in this book for you. I know it's great advice, because I've used it myself, and I've seen it in practice time and time again. It's the same thing I tell clients when I consult with them, and when I get on the phone with them.

I have no problem giving advice over the phone, and I'm not one of those guys who charges just for a phone call. But what I will do in the call is give suggestions, and expect to see them implemented. When you read this book, I have no way of checking into whether you're implementing what I suggest. I can just tell you that you have no way of seeing how it works unless you put it into action.

I know very well that there are a lot of physical therapists, physicians, dentists, spinal surgeons, etc. out there who don't see the need for this because they've always done it a certain way. But I assure you that changing your mindset, how you practice, and how you conduct your business will be substantially worthwhile for you. Even if we just change things 10% in each area, that's going to end up being a 30% growth. That will be huge for your bottom line. And if we start down that road, I can guarantee your business will look different—in a good way—by day two.

It's all about mindset—and too many of us practitioners never develop the mindset we need because we don't discover we need it until too late. Medical school is about medicine, but once we are running our own practices, a large proportion of our time (for some of us, almost all of it) will be spent as a businessperson. We don't need years in school for that, but we do need the right mindset. We need to be ready to promote ourselves and to constantly think about the health of our businesses as much as we do the health of our patients.

Without that ingredient, nothing can happen. If you're not ready to work on your practice more than you work in it, nothing I tell you in this book can help you. The only reason most medical professionals struggle in business is they are unwilling to see themselves as

Dr. Joseph Simon

businesspeople. Make that mindset shift, and you're already way ahead of the game.

Remember You're In Business

Do you know the difference between a proprietor and an entrepreneur? What about the difference between marketing and sales? You may think you do, but the fact is being a medical practitioner and being the best at what you do doesn't always leave you a lot of time to learn how to work on your practice rather than in your practice, let alone to implement what you learn.

Your practice is a business. All practices are. And more people are realizing that they need to be run that way. It's a revolution that's happening slowly, but it's spreading to more and more people. Most practitioners still don't realize that, though, and if you do, that gives you an automatic edge. They still think, "I have a professional title. I have professional training. I'm respected in the community. If I hang my shingle outside, everyone will beat down my door." It's not true anymore, and that's becoming ever clearer.

Most practitioners I talk to instinctively hate that. They don't want to be business owners. They don't want to be salespeople. They'd rather outsource that. I understand. In fact, I'm generally a big proponent of outsourcing, as you'll find out. But one has to do it intelligently, and you can't outsource the captain of the ship. If you hire somebody else to be in charge, they're going to be less motivated because they're collecting a salary no matter what, and they're going to run things their own way—good or bad—because you gave them the power to do it.

176

But the fact that you're reading this now means you're willing to learn to be a businessperson even though they didn't teach it in medical or dental school. You're willing to be your own captain; that will help you a lot. If you want your practice to succeed, you can't just let success come to you. It's true that everyone needs healthcare, but you can't just assume as a cash-based practice that everyone is going to need it from *you*. The advice I've given in this book is real and the strategies are practical and actionable ones that you can use to grow your practice and keep it successful.

I've long appreciated the work of business guru Dan Kennedy, who made the very important point that in a certain sense, all businesses are the same. As a business owner, you have the same goals as all the other business owners out there: to bring in clients who will pay for what you do, and to keep them coming back. In other words, all businesses are in the business of marketing. And they all need to have systems in place to make sure that happens as effectively as it can.

Keep your mind on the purpose of your practice: it's to generate money, and to build something that will remain for the next generation. To do that, you need to get paid well, as you deserve to be, for the skills you've acquired as a medical professional, and you need to develop new skills as a businessperson in order to make that happen.

Running a private practice, it's going to be imperative for you to have or develop management skills. Chances are you didn't get these when you got your medical training, or if you did, they were very rudimentary. When I was in college, we didn't get business training at all. Now I'm starting to hear that it's changing a little, but very slowly.

Personally, I have a lot of students come into my practice, and when they do, I can tell right off the bat which ones really want to get their hands dirty and find out firsthand how a private clinic is run, and which ones just want to pass their affiliation or clinical and go on to a day job.

Since you're looking to have a private practice and probably move away from or keep from having to go back to a day job, you don't want to be in that second group of students. I get a lot of students in my practice who are ready to jump into anything and want to start their own practice right out of the gate. You might or might not be a student like that, but to get everything from this book, you'll want to capture that same drive that they have.

When I helped my wife start her practice, we talked to a lot of her friends from medical school. They're brilliant; they're some of the smartest people I know. And they love the fact that they've graduated medical school in a field they love, and that now they get to help patients. But they're baffled by the fact that a small business owner down the street who didn't even go to college may be making three times what they make.

So, yes. You get the honor and reputation of being a doctor no matter what. And if that's all you want, then great. Running a practice isn't for a person like that. But you need to be a businessperson if you want financial freedom. Because no matter how much money you make when you work for someone else, you end up living paycheck to paycheck.

Entrepreneurs control their own destinies. It's true in all industries. The people I know who have left big companies are now making more money running their own cupcake shops than they were as financial analysts.

I think it all comes down to two things, and if you can do them, you have the most important tools you need for success: having ideas and implementing those ideas. I meet practitioners every day who have plenty of amazing ideas but can never get them implemented.

That's true for marketing ideas, business ideas, product ideas, and everything you can imagine. These can all jumpstart your practice, but you have to make them happen. And that doesn't always happen overnight. It can be harder for a lot of us because we've been trained to work for a business and never on a business—which is just what we need to do if we want to be successful.

I hope to give you plenty of ideas that work well and that can help stir your creative energies to come up with ideas of your own. I hope to inspire you to put those ideas into action as well.

The $70,000 Gift

That kind of resourcefulness is integral to what I call my $70,000 gift. It's something that comes up when I consult with practitioners. When they first sign on, one of the things that they naturally want to know is whether I can make them back the money they're spending on hiring me.

I charge a lot of money, but I guarantee my clients they can get their money back in the first month. If I can't make them back that money, I refund everything they paid me. Which really makes it a no-lose situation for them. But often they can't believe it. They look at how much they're making now and don't believe it can go up by that much.

But for me, it's very simple. It's something anyone could do. It comes down to going back to the methods I outlined earlier. Go to your database and print out your e-mail list. Print out demographics. Do it for every patient that you have. Figure out their age, male/female ratio, and their ZIP code. Save the data from those three things, and then figure out what they make. You probably don't have the exact numbers on it, but you can usually take a pretty good guess based on occupation.

If there a university or a big company close by, that gives you an even better idea of people's possible occupations and pay scales, and an even better opportunity to narrow your marketing approach to them.

Based on that you can now do Facebook campaigns and mailers, and you can even do every-door direct mail with the post office, since you now have the ZIP codes and know where your patients are coming from.

You can now do simple "reactivation" campaigns. That means a letter to your old patients updating them on what's going on now with your practice and explaining why they should come back.

You can do a referral campaign asking them to send a friend or family member in, maybe in exchange for some kind of deal on their own rate.

The possibilities are infinite as far as things that you can come up with based on that information that you already have access to. The gold is truly sitting in those charts. And that's what a lot of my clients don't realize when they pay me that $70,000 challenge.

Then they start to realize after that first month that the money is really coming in—and after the second and third it still is. Often we discover that you can run campaigns based on those same lists month after month the whole year round, especially since the patient databases at a lot of offices have an unbelievably massive amount of data.

Sometimes there are just so many names that as a practical matter you just can't market to them all at once. You have to break it up. Do just the last six month, or go back two or five years. It's a resource that truly keeps renewing itself.

And that's why I call it the $70,000 gift. Over the course of several months, the income generated from the campaign easily generates $70,000.

Closing Remarks

At the end of the day, I ask my business partners, clients, and friends the same question: why? Why do we care so much about our practices? Why do we care so much about the wellbeing of other people (not just our patients but staff as well)? Why do we still offer our services, knowing that we might not get paid for our time and expertise. In my opinion, as leaders, we are built a certain way.

In the United States, the common misconception among patients is that I have insurance and that should take care of everything. Nine out of ten patients do not know their own health insurance details.

I challenge you to survey your patients today and quiz them about the details of their own insurance plans. Ask to see if they understand the difference between a copay, coinsurance, and deductible. The results might surprise you. So I implore you not to look at your practice as a commoditized service. Look at it as a value driven offer that will help your patients achieve the results they desire, but also as a bridge between you and your patients' understanding of their insurance plan.

I know you care about your patients. I want you to create a business that will not only create financial success for you and your staff, but also be able to deliver that value and expertise down to your patients.

So as I stated in this book multiple times, it would be a disservice to your patients, your community, and your profession if you don't advertise, market, and educate the general public about the benefits of your services. I created the Private Practice Business Academy to help practitioners like yourself to have a place to learn, share, and explore the business aspects of their private practice.

It takes time and dedication to run and grow a business. A medical practice is no different (except we deal with people suffering in pain). I hope you take a moment to apply the lessons of this book into your own practice today. To continue your business education you can go to privatepracticebusinessacademy.com to sign up to receive my insights through my podcast.

Your practice should be exactly what you envisioned on day one. Let me help you see that vision again.

"Change your marketing. Change your results. Change your practice"

– @DrJoeSimon

ABOUT THE AUTHOR

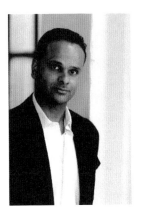

Dr. Joe Simon is a husband and a father of two (four if counting his furkids). He's been a private practice owner & practitioner for 15+ years, and is perpetually in pursuit of multiple entrepreneurial endeavors within the health and wellness fields. One thing that keeps his passion and drive strong is the opportunity to not just treat patients, but also help physicians, dentists, acupuncturists, chiropractors, physical therapists, fitness professionals, etc. develop or extend their business models, marketing strategies, and growth / exit plans.

He has a deep passion for creating, marketing, and growing a private practice and believes that if you follow the right formula, anyone can be successful. To date, over 15,000 Physical Therapists, 550 physician practices, and 20 hospitals worldwide (US, Canada, Europe) have benefited from his business, management, and marketing techniques.

55349822R00108

Made in the USA
Charleston, SC
21 April 2016